ISBN: 9781073890934

30-DAY
QUICK DIET
For Men

Gail Johnson, M.S.
Ron Hill, Jr.

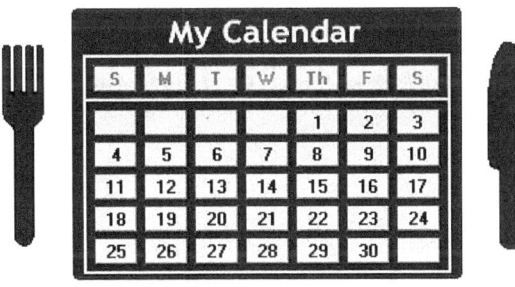

NoPaperPress™

CONTENTS

The Best Weight-Loss Diets (6)
Begin with a Medical Exam
What's in This book? (6)
Which Calorie Level is for You?
How Much Weight Will You Lose? (7)
Guidelines for Healthy Eating
Exchanging Foods (9)
Two Nights Off
Frozen Dinners (10)
Eating Out
Quick Diet Info (11)
Important Notes

1500 CALORIE MEAL PLANS
Day 1 to Day 5   (14)
Day 6 to Day 10 (19)
Day 11 to Day 15 (24)
Day 16 to Day 20 (29)
Day 21 to Day 25 (34)
Day 26 to Day 30 (39)

1800 CALORIE MEAL PLANS
Day 1 to Day 5 (45)
Day 6 to Day 10 (50)
Day 11 to Day 15 (55)
Day 16 to Day 20 (60)
Day 21 to Day 25 (65)
Day 26 to Day 30 (70)

RECIPIES & DIET TIPS
Day 1 Recipe: Baked Herb-Crusted Cod (76)
Day 2 Recipe: French-Toasted English Muffin
Day 3 Recipe: Chicken with Peppers & Onions (78)
Day 4 Recipe: Meat Loaf
Day 5 Recipe: Frozen-Fish Dinner (80)
Day 6 Recipe: Grandma's Pizza
Day 7 Recipe: Chicken Dinner - Out (82)
Day 8 Recipe: Baked Salmon with Salsa
Day 9 Recipe: Veggie Burger (84)
Day 10 Recipe: Wild-Blueberry Pancakes (85)

Day 11 Recipe: Artichoke-Bean Salad
Day 12 Recipe: Fish Dinner - Out (87)
Day 13 Recipe: Pasta with Marinara Sauce
Day 14 Recipe: Oatena Cereal Mix (89)
Day 15 Recipe: London Broil
Day 16 Recipe: Baked Red Snapper (91)
Day 17 Recipe: Cajun Chicken Salad
Day 18 Recipe: Grilled Swordfish (93)
Day 19 Recipe: Chinese Dinner - Out
Day 20 Recipe: Quick Pasta alla Puttanesca (95)
Day 21 Recipe: Frozen-Meat Dinner
Day 22 Recipe: Shrimp & Spinach Salad (97)
Day 23 Recipe: Beans & Greens Salad
Day 24 Recipe: Four Bean Plus Salad (99)
Day 25 Recipe: Hanger Steak
Day 26 Recipe: Grilled Scallops & Polenta (101)
Day 27 Recipe: Fettuccine in Summer Sauce
Day 28 Recipe: Frozen Chicken Dinner (103)
Day 29 Recipe: Barbequed Shrimp
Day 30 Recipe: Cheeseburger (105)

Appendix A Frozen Foods (106)

Appendix B Frozen Food Safety (112)

Appendix C Soup Selections (113)

NoPaperPress Paperbacks & eBooks (114)

Disclaimer

The Best Weight-Loss Diets

According to the late Dr. Jean Mayer of Harvard University's Department of Nutrition, a really good weight-loss diet must have the following three characteristics:

1) The diet must provide you with an understanding of weight control as well as the knowledge you need to reduce your weight to the desired level.

2) The diet must help you remain healthy while you are losing weight.

3) The diet must lead you to a healthier way of eating and exercising that will, in the long term, help you keep off the weight you have lost.

The weight-loss diet featured in this book is a "balanced diet;" i.e., a diet that is not only low calorie and reasonably low in fat, but is also nutritionally balanced. The *30-Day Quick Diet for Men*, however, does not meet all the criteria set forth above. While you will get some "dieting insight" and some idea of how much you can eat and still lose weight, you will not get a real understanding of weight control from this book. That's not its purpose. What you will get is a healthy diet – and a diet that if followed will promote weight loss. Think of the *30-Day Quick Diet* as a quick fix, a healthy start that will get you on the right track – but it's not the long-term answer.

Long-term success is about developing both an understanding and a plan that will result in healthier eating and physical activity habits. For a through understanding and the guidance you need to succeed in the long term I recommend you read, *Weight Control - U.S. Edition* by Vincent Antonetti, Ph.D., a NoPaperPress book.

Begin with a Medical Exam

Everyone should at the very least have a medical assessment, or exam, before starting a weight loss diet. Why? You need to make sure your health will allow you to lower your caloric intake and increase your physical activity. The medical checkup may be as simple as a visit to a physician who is familiar with your medical history, or it may be a thorough physical exam. The physician conducting the medical exam should be made aware of and should approve the specific weight loss diet you're planning.

What's in This Book?

This book actually contains two 30-day diets: an 1800 Calorie diet, and for even faster weight loss a 1500 Calorie diet. And both diets have a meal plan (menu) for each and every one of the 30 days.

Which Calorie Level is for You?
1500 Calorie Quick Diet: Smaller men, older men and inactive men should select this calorie level.
1800 Calorie Quick Diet: This calorie level is only for larger men, younger men and active men.

How Much Weight Will You Lose?
Weight loss occurs when your food energy intake is less than the total energy you expend. This difference in calories is referred to as your calorie deficit. How much weight you lose depends on the magnitude of your calorie deficit. Simple metabolic calculations make a rough estimate possible. **On the 30-Day Quick Diet, most men lose 15 to 20 pounds** – depending on whether the 1,800 or 1,500 Calorie diet is selected. Smaller men, older men and less active men will lose a bit less and larger men, younger men and more active men often much more. Exactly how much weight you will lose depends on how much you weigh, your age and your activity level. Again, for the full story see *Weight Control - U.S. Edition* by Vincent Antonetti, Ph.D.

Guidelines for Healthy Eating
No single food can supply all the nutrients you need in the amounts you need. The most important factors in nutrition are variety, variety, variety! **Variety is the key to a nutritious diet.** As a means of setting strategies for food selection, the U.S. Department of Health and Human Services and the Department of Agriculture issue Dietary Guidelines every five years. The latest Dietary Guidelines describe a healthy diet as one that:
- Emphasizes fruits, vegetables, whole grains, and fat-free or low-fat milk products.
- Includes fish, poultry, lean meats, beans and nuts.
- Is low in saturated fats, trans fats, cholesterol, salt (sodium) and added sugars.

      The guidelines encourage adults to consume a variety of nutrient-dense foods and beverages within their caloric needs. In 2005, the afore mentioned U.S. government agencies recommended how much should be eaten from each of the basic food groups (i.e., from the fruit group, vegetable group, grains group, meat and beans group, milk group, and oils group) to meet your caloric goal – whether you are trying to lose weight or maintain weight. All this information and more can be found in our book Eat Smart - *U.S. Edition* published by NoPaperPress.

Even though most adults can get all the vitamins and minerals they need by merely consuming a variety of nutritious foods (from the fruit group, the vegetable group, the grains group, the meat and beans group, the milk group, and the oils group), many physicians recommend a daily multi-vitamin/mineral supplement – just in case you don't eat the way you should.

Large Green Salad: One of the dinner mainstays is a "Large Green Salad." Prepare your "Large Green Salad" in a bowl with a volume of at least 16 ounces, or 2 cups. First add about 1 cup of either green leaf lettuce, Romaine lettuce or a mesclun mix. Then add, as desired, half cup of green veggies such as broccoli, celery, cucumber, peppers, spinach, or watercress. This vegetable combination will, on average, total about 35 Calories. You will be eating a "Large Green Salad" just about every day at dinnertime. Remember that variety is the key to a nutritious diet. So be sure to vary the ingredients of the salad.

Top your "Large Green Salad" with 1½ tablespoons of any light salad dressing available at your local supermarket that contains no more than 25 Calories per tablespoon. Some of our favorite light salad dressings are:
  - **Ken's Steakhouse Fat Free Raspberry Pecan**
  - **Kraft Light Done Right House Italian**
  - **Wishbone Just 2 Good Honey Dijon**
  - **Newman's Lighten Up! Balsamic Vinaigrette**
Your "Large Green Salad" with salad dressing will cost you roughly 70 Calories but will be packed with lots of health-giving vitamins, minerals and fiber.

About Bread: First understand that bread, more specifically whole-grain breads, are good sources of complex carbohydrates and dietary fiber, as well as several B vitamins (thiamin, riboflavin, niacin, and foliate), vitamin E, and minerals (iron, magnesium and selenium). In recent years, however, sliced bread loaves have gotten larger, as have the bread slices inside these loaves. Just a few years ago the standard slice of bread contained about 65 to 70 Calories – now most are 100 plus Calories.

The *30-Day Quick Diet* requires whole-grain bread at 65 to 70 Calories per slice. Quite a few bakers sell thin sliced or "light" sliced bread. The difficult part is finding a whole grain thin sliced or "light" bread (with about 70 Calories per slice). Whatever the brand, make sure the first word in the Ingredients list is "whole." "Pepperidge Farm Small Slice 100% Whole Wheat" is a good choice. It's whole grain, has 70 Calories per slice and it tastes good too.

Exchanging Foods

If there is a food listed in the *30-Day Quick Diet* that you don't like, or perhaps that you forgot to pick up while shopping, you probably can exchange or substitute another food in its place – a technique used by dieticians. Exchanging a food listed in a diet for another food with approximately equal caloric value and nutritional content is the foundation of a successful long-term diet. Substitution possibilities are almost endless but have to be done carefully.

The easiest substitutions are those within the same food group, such as exchanging one vegetable variety for another, or a glass of milk for a cup of yogurt. More sophisticated exchanges cross food groups, for instance replacing 3½ ounces of turkey with a tablespoon of peanut butter spread on a piece of whole wheat bread. Both foods are complete protein and both contain about 175 Calories.

Refer to a good online calorie table. With some understanding and experience, you can use this table to help you substitute foods called for in the *30-Day Quick Diet* with equal calorie foods from the same food group.

Breakfast: You may substitute any cereal for any other wholesome cereal. For example, if you're not crazy about having Shredded Wheat for breakfast on Day 6, substitute Wheat Chex or Cheerios, etc. If you don't like the soft-boiled egg called for on Day 9, make yourself a scrambled egg instead. And if Cantaloupe is on the menu but is not in season, replace the cantaloupe with a half cup of orange juice.

Snacks: Again, where yogurt is specified you may substitute an 8-ounce glass of skim milk, but to maintain a nutritionally balanced diet keep this snack a dairy selection. Similarly, when fruit is on the agenda, you may select another type of fruit but do not stray from the fruit group. Nuts and popcorn can be interchanged at will. (Incidentally, you should buy a hot-air popper. They make great popcorn – which is high in fiber and makes a tasty and nutritious snack.)

Two Nights Off

Everyone deserves a break from the grind of preparing dinner after coming home from work. So the *30-Day Quick Diet* gives you two days off per week! Notice that one night a week the meal plan calls for a frozen dinner and on a second night during the week you're encouraged to eat out. There are, however, some rules and caveats involved and these are covered in the next two sections.

Frozen Dinners

In general, a frozen dinner should not be a meal in itself. Make sure you add a salad, fruit, bread etc. The frozen dinner you choose should come with at least one cup of cooked vegetables. If your frozen dinner doesn't measure up, add your own frozen, fresh or canned vegetables. And look for dinners with no more than 800 mg of sodium. In addition, make sure the dinner you choose has no more than 30 percent of the daily value for total fat. **Appendix A** (page 106) lists almost 150 frozen dinner entrees.

And on the days when a frozen dinner is specified, you will also be given a calorie goal for the frozen dinner. For example, Day 5 calls for frozen fish dinner with a maximum allowable 300 Calories. If you choose a frozen fish dinner that contains less than 300 Calories, you may spend the unused calories any way you wish.

Moreover, on those nights when you just don't have the energy or time to cook, you can always substitute a frozen dinner for the entree listed in the meal plan. For example, Day 1 calls for Herb-Crusted Cod for dinner. The total calorie count for dinner is 525. In place of the cod, any combination of a frozen fish dinner and side dishes (salads, etc) with a total calorie content close to 525 would be an acceptable, albeit not as tasty, an alternative.

Eating Out

You may eat out once a week. When you're on a diet, however, eating in a restaurant can be a challenge, because most restaurant portions are huge, and can easily total more than 1,000 Calories. On the *30-Day Quick Diet*, a dinner type (i.e., fish, chicken, etc) and a calorie target is specified. For example Day 7 of the 1,500 Calorie diet specifies a chicken dinner and allows you 630 Calories.

First, you need to choose a restaurant where you have a fighting chance to achieve your calorie goal. Next, order simple, such as broiled fish with steamed vegetables and brown rice. Tell the waiter you want no sauce, no gravy, nothing added. Then, knowing your calorie objective, and that most fish and chicken are about 50 Calories per ounce, most steamed vegetable servings average approximately 50 Calories per cup, and rice is about 100 Calories per ½ cup, decide how much to eat – and take the remainder home. If fresh fruit is not an option, pass on dessert and have the evening snack specified in the meal plan for that day.

Quick Diet Info

As mentioned previously, there are two diet plans in this book:

-.1500 Calorie 30-Day Diet starts on page 14.
- 1800 Calorie 30-Day Diet starts on page 45.
Both have a detailed meal plan for each of the 30 days. Associated with each day is a "Recipe of the Day" and a "Diet Tip of the Day."

Both the 1500 and 1800 Calorie diets adhere to the United States Department of Agriculture recommendation that suggest a balanced diet should have approximately 50 percent of its calories from carbs, about 20 percent from protein sources and 30 percent or less from fat. (Note, the *30-Day Quick Diet* may not be appropriate for individuals with illnesses such as heart disease, diabetes, food allergies, etc. Again, please see your physician before starting any diet.)

After you complete the 30th day on the diet, if you still want to lose more weight a good alternative is to repeat the diet by starting over at Day1.

Important Notes

1) Coffee may be decaf or regular. If desired, skim milk and a sugar substitute may be added to coffee or tea. And soy and almond milk may be used instead of cow's milk.

2) Fried eggs or scrambled eggs should be cooked in a pan coated with a non-stick cooking spray. Hard-boiled eggs may be substituted for fried, scrambled or soft-boiled eggs.

3) Cereals should be whole grain and unsweetened. At the top of the list are Old-fashioned Oatmeal, Wheatena and Shredded Wheat. Among other reasonably healthy choices are Cheerios, Wheat Chex, Wheaties, some Kashi cereals and Farina. When blueberries are in season, you may add blueberries instead of raisins to your cereal. (Substitution ratio = 2 blueberries per raisin.)

4) Bread may be either plain or toasted whole grain, such as whole wheat, whole rye or pumpernickel. Look for whole grain varieties that contain 70 Calories per slice. If desired, bread may be sprayed with a zero-calorie butter substitute. NO BUTTER!

5) When soup in a microwaveable bowl is specified, eat only one serving (8 ounces) unless otherwise noted. (Microwaveable bowls usually contain about two servings.)

6) Use freely as desired: clear unsweetened coffee, clear unsweetened tea, water, seltzer water and any diet soda, clear soups without fat, bouillon, and seasonings such as mustard, cinnamon, dill, herbs, red and black pepper, curry, vinegar, lemon juice and sections, and dill and sour pickles.

7) Use only lean cuts of meat trimmed of all visible fat. Poultry should be limited to chicken or turkey breasts (white meat only and skinless).

8) When canned tuna or salmon is specified, use only fish packed in water.

9) When the diet calls for turkey bacon, make sure the brand you buy has no more than 35 Calories per slice.

10) An unlimited amount of green salad may be eaten, but the salad dressing should be as specified.

11) Use freely as desired: clear unsweetened coffee, clear unsweetened tea, water, seltzer, any diet soda, clear soups without fat, bouillon, and seasonings such as mustard, cinnamon, dill, herbs, red and black pepper, curry, vinegar, lemon juice and sections, and dill and sour pickles.

12) If it's more convenient, any food item may be moved to any part of the day and combined with any meal or snack.

13) If you cannot find the exact item called for in the diet (because it's out of stock or discontinued), substitute a comparable food (of the same type and close caloric value).

14) Although it's recommended that you follow the diet days as specified, it's fine to occasionally skip a day and/or pick and choose the days you prefer. (Nutritionally, each day stands on its own.)

1500-Calorie
Daily Menus

Day 1 – 1500 Calorie Meal Plan

BREAKFAST	Calories	Totals
Orange juice (½ cup)	50	
Wheaties (¾ cup) + ½ cup skim milk + ½ banana	190	
Whole-grain toast (1 slice) (See page 8)	65	
Coffee (See **Notes** - page 11)	10	315 Cal
SNACK		
Fresh fruit in season (apple, peach, etc)	70	
Coffee or tea	10	80 Cal
LUNCH		
Soup (Appendix C - page 113)	110	
Turkey breast (1 oz) on 1 slice rye bread	105	
Pickle spear	0	
Lettuce & tomato slices	20	
Coffee or tea	10	245 Cal
SNACK		
Two small cookies (See note bottom Day 3 Daily Menu)	160	
Skim milk (6 oz)	60	220 Cal
DINNER		
Baked Herb-Crusted Cod (Day 1 Recipe - page 76)	230	
Spinach (½ cup) steamed with garlic & drizzled	100	
Asparagus (7 spear cooked & drained)	20	
Baked potato (medium)	100	
Whole grain bread (1 slice)	65	
Water with lemon wedge	15	530 Cal
SNACK		
Popcorn Mini Bag*	110	110 Cal
* Such as Orville Redenbacher's Smart Pop.		1500 Cal

14

Day 2 – 1500 Calorie Meal Plan

BREAKFAST	Calories	Totals
Fresh or frozen strawberries (½ cup)	25	
French toasted English Muffin (Day 2 Recipe - page 77)	270	
Light syrup (1 Tbsp)	30	
Coffee	10	335 Cal
SNACK		
Yogurt (6 oz, nonfat, any flavor)	90	
Coffee or tea	10	100 Cal
LUNCH		
Salad (3 oz tuna, 1 tsp Evoo, onions & celery)	175	
Lettuce & tomato wedges	20	
Rye bread (1 slice)	65	
Fresh fruit in season (apple, plum, etc)	70	
Coffee or tea	10	340 Cal
SNACK		
Handful unsalted mixed nuts	100	
Coffee or tea	10	110 Cal
DINNER		
Broiled veal chop (4 oz lean)	200	
Corn on the cob (1 medium ear)	100	
Broccoli (½ cup steamed & drizzled with 1 tsp	70	
Large green salad with 1½ Tbsp low-cal dressing*	70	
Hot or iced tea	10	450 Cal
SNACK		
Graham crackers (4 squares)	120	
Skim milk (4 oz)	45	165 Cal
* See Large Green Salad - page 8.		**1500 Cal**

Day 3 – 1500 Calorie Meal Plan

BREAKFAST	Calories	Totals
Grapefruit (½)	75	
Scrambled egg (See **Notes** - page 11)	80	
Turkey bacon (1 slice)	35	
Whole grain toast (1 slice)	65	
Coffee	10	265 Cal
SNACK		
Yogurt (6 oz, nonfat, any flavor)	90	
Coffee or tea	10	100 Cal
LUNCH		
Ham (2 oz) with mustard on 2 slices rye bread	290	
Pickle spear	0	
Small bunch of grapes	65	
Gelatin dessert (unsweetened)	10	
Diet soda or water	0	365 Cal
SNACK		
Popcorn Mini Bag	110	110 Cal
DINNER		
Chicken w Peppers & Onions (Day 3 Recipe - page 78)	250	
For preparation remaining food - see Day 3 Recipe	70	
Whole-grain bread (1 slice)	65	
Fresh fruit in season (apple, peach, etc))	70	
Water	0	575 Cal
SNACK		
One small cookie*	80	
Coffee or tea	10	90 Cal
* Oatmeal, ginger snap, sugar, etc - check calories!		1500 Cal

Day 4 – 1500 Calorie Meal Plan

BREAKFAST	Calories	Totals
Grapefruit (½)	75	
Cheerios (1 cup) + ½ cup skim milk + about 15 raisins*	190	
Coffee	10	275 Cal
SNACK		
Fresh fruit in season (apple, peach, etc)	70	
Coffee or tea	10	80 Cal
LUNCH		
Subway 6" (Ham, Cheese + veggies)*	260	
Canned pineapple (1 cup, no-sugar-added juice)	80	
Water with lemon wedge	10	350 Cal
* On 6" half wheat roll.		
SNACK		
Handful unsalted mixed nuts	100	
Coffee or tea	10	110 Cal
DINNER		
Meat Loaf (Day 4 Recipe - page 79)	290	
One-half acorn squash (baked with ½ tsp maple	90	
Spinach (½ cup steamed & drizzled with 1 tsp	70	
Romaine lettuce, tomato slices & 1 Tbsp low-cal	45	
Gelatin dessert (unsweetened)	10	
Hot or iced tea	10	515 Cal
SNACK		
Two small Ginger Snap cookies	160	
Coffee or tea	10	170 Cal
* See **Notes** - page 11 re substituting blueberries for raisins.		1500 Cal

Day 5 – 1500 Calorie Meal Plan

BREAKFAST	Calories	Totals
Cantaloupe (½ medium)	50	
Fried egg	80	
Toasted raisin bread (1 slice)	75	
Coffee	10	215 Cal
SNACK		
Yogurt (6 oz, nonfat, any flavor)	90	
Coffee or tea	10	100 Cal
LUNCH		
Soup (Appendix C - page 113)	140	
Small whole-grain roll	80	
Lettuce and sliced tomato with 1 Tbsp low-cal	45	
Canned pineapple (½ cup, no-sugar-added juice)	40	
Hot or iced tea	10	315 Cal
SNACK		
Popcorn Mini Bag	110	
Coffee or tea	10	120 Cal
DINNER		
Frozen fish dinner (Day 5 Recipe - page 80)	340	
Large green salad with 1½ Tbsp low-cal dressing	70	
Whole-grain bread (1 slice)	65	
Fresh fruit in season (apple, peach, etc)	70	
Water with lemon wedge	15	560 Cal
SNACK		
Graham crackers (4 squares)	120	
Skim milk (6 oz)	70	190 Cal
		1500 Cal

Day 6 – 1500 Calorie Meal Plan

BREAKFAST	Calories	Totals
Tomato juice (½ cup)	20	
Shredded Wheat (1 cup) + ½ cup skim milk + ½ banana	265	
Coffee	10	295 Cal
SNACK		
Handful unsalted mixed nuts	100	
Coffee or tea	10	110 Cal
LUNCH		
Leftover meat loaf (½ Day 4 serving size with ketchup)	155	
Small whole-grain roll	80	
Lettuce	0	
Fresh or frozen berries (½ cup)	50	
Hot or iced tea	10	295 Cal
SNACK		
Yogurt (6 oz, nonfat, any flavor)	90	
Coffee or tea	10	100 Cal
DINNER		
Pizza (Day 6 Recipe - page 81)	350	
Large green salad with 1½ Tbsp low-cal dressing	70	
Fresh fruit in season (peach, plum, etc)	70	
Glass of red wine (4 oz)	100	
Hot or iced tea	10	600 Cal
SNACK		
Graham Crackers (3 squares)	90	
Coffee or tea	10	100 Cal
		1500 Cal

Day 7 – 1500 Calorie Meal Plan

BREAKFAST	Calories	Totals
Cantaloupe (½ medium)	50	
Oatmeal (½ cup dry) + ½ cup skim milk + about 15 raisins	220	
Coffee	10	280 Cal
SNACK		
Fresh fruit in season (pear, plum, etc)	70	70 Cal
LUNCH		
Soup (Appendix C - page 113)	100	
Grilled cheese sandwich (2 slices 2% cheese)	230	
Lettuce and sliced tomato	20	
Pickle spear	0	
Water	0	350 Cal
SNACK		
Carrot sticks + ¼ cup low-fat cottage cheese & chives	60	
Coffee or tea	10	70 Cal
DINNER		
Eat Out – Chicken dinner (Day 7 Recipe - page 82)		
Max allowable calories	630	630 Cal
	0	
SNACK		
Graham crackers (3 squares)	90	
Coffee or tea	10	100 Cal
		1500 Cal

Day 8 – 1500 Calorie Meal Plan

BREAKFAST	Calories	Totals
Cantaloupe (½ medium)	50	
Wheaties (¾ cup) + ½ cup skim milk + ½ banana	190	
Whole-grain toast (1 slice)	65	
Coffee	10	315 Cal
SNACK		
Fresh fruit in season (apple, peach, etc)	70	
Coffee or tea	10	80 Cal
LUNCH		
Chorizo, Egg & Cheese*	260	
Hot or iced tea	10	270 Cal
* Hot Pockets (wrap) or if unavailable an equivalent food.		
SNACK		
Two small cookies	160	
Skim milk (4 oz)	410	200 Cal
DINNER		
Baked salmon with salsa (Day 8 Recipe - page 83)	215	
Summer squash, zucchini and tomatoes	60	
Brown rice (½ cup)	100	
Large green salad with 1½ Tbsp low-cal dressing	70	
Fresh fruit in season (apple, plum, etc)	70	
Water with lemon wedge	15	515 Cal
SNACK		
Popcorn Mini Bag	110	
Coffee or tea	10	120 Cal
		1500 Cal

Day 9 – 1500 Calorie Meal Plan

BREAKFAST	Calories	Totals
Orange juice (½ cup)	50	
Soft-boiled (or poached) egg	80	
Whole-grain toast (2 slices)	130	
Coffee	10	270 Cal
SNACK		
Yogurt (6 oz, nonfat, any flavor)	90	
Coffee or tea	10	100 Cal
LUNCH		
Salad (3 oz tuna, 1 tsp Evoo, onions & celery)	175	
Lettuce & tomato wedges + rye bread (1 slice)	85	
Fresh fruit in season – (apple, pear, etc)	70	
Gelatin dessert (unsweetened)	10	
Coffee or tea	10	350 Cal
SNACK		
Handful unsalted mixed nuts	100	
Coffee or tea	10	110 Cal
DINNER		
Veggie burger – (1 patty) (Day 9 Recipe - page 84)	100	
Low-fat cheddar cheese (1 thin slice)	50	
Beets (3 small) + Seeded hamburger roll	185	
Large green salad with 1½ Tbsp low-cal dressing	70	
Fresh fruit in season (apple, peach, etc)	70	
Hot or iced tea	10	485 Cal
SNACK		
Graham crackers (4 squares)	120	
Skim milk (6 oz)	60	180 Cal
		1495 Cal

Day 10 – 1500 Calorie Meal Plan

BREAKFAST	Calories	Totals
Orange juice (½ cup)	50	
Wild blueberry pancakes (Day 10 Recipe - page 85)	190	
Turkey bacon (2 slices)	70	
Light syrup (1½ Tbsp)	45	
Coffee	10	365 Cal
SNACK		
Yogurt (6 oz, nonfat, any flavor)	90	
Coffee or tea	10	100 Cal
LUNCH		
Peanut butter (2 Tbsp) on 2 slices of whole-grain bread	330	
Skim milk (4 oz)	45	
Fresh fruit in season (apple, peach, etc)	70	445 Cal
SNACK		
Handful of mixed unsalted nuts	100	100 Cal
DINNER		
Broiled pork chop (about ½" thick trimmed of fat)	260	
Green peas (½ cup)	55	
Tomato & cucumber salad 2 Tbsp low-cal dressing	70	
Hot or iced tea	10	395 Cal
SNACK		
Fiber One Chocolate Fudge Brownie	90	
Coffee or tea	10	100 Cal
		1505 Cal

Day 11 – 1500 Calorie Meal Plan

BREAKFAST	Calories	Totals
Fresh sliced orange	75	
Cheerios (1 cup) + ½ cup skim milk + about 15 raisins	190	
Whole grain toast (1 slice)	65	
Coffee	10	340 Cal
SNACK		
Fresh fruit in season (pear, plum, etc)	70	
Coffee or tea	10	80 Cal
LUNCH		
Cottage cheese (1 cup low fat)	180	
Large green salad with 1½ Tbsp low-cal dressing	70	
Small whole-grain roll	80	
Hot or iced tea	10	340 Cal
SNACK		
Handful unsalted mixed nuts	100	
Coffee or tea	10	110 Cal
DINNER		
Grilled chicken sausage (2 links about 2½ oz per link)	180	
Artichoke-bean salad (Day 11 Recipe - page 86)	190	
Green beans - steamed	25	
Whole-grain bread (1 slice)	65	
Hot or iced tea	10	470 Cal
SNACK		
Two small cookies	160	
Coffee or tea	10	170 Cal
		1510 Cal

Day 12 – 1500 Calorie Meal Plan

BREAKFAST	Calories	Totals
Grapefruit (½)	75	
Scrambled egg	80	
Turkey bacon (2 slices)	70	
Whole-grain toast (1 slice)	65	
Coffee	10	300 Cal
SNACK		
Yogurt (6 oz, nonfat, any flavor)	90	
Coffee or tea	10	100 Cal
LUNCH		
Soup (Appendix C - page 113)	160	
Tomato slices (¼ cup chopped fresh basil + 1 tsp Evoo)	60	
Whole-grain bread (1 slice)	65	
Gelatin dessert (unsweetened)	10	
Hot or iced tea	10	305 Cal
SNACK		
Fresh fruit in season (apple, plum, etc)	70	70 Cal
DINNER		
Eat Out – Fish dinner (Day 12 Recipe - page 87)		
Max allowable calories	595	595 Cal
	0	
SNACK		
Graham crackers (4 squares)	120	
Coffee or tea	10	130 Cal
		1500 Cal

Day 13 – 1500 Calorie Meal Plan

BREAKFAST	Calories	Totals
Orange juice (½ cup)	50	
Shredded Wheat (1 cup) + ½ cup skim milk + ½ banana	260	
Coffee	10	320 Cal
SNACK		
Handful unsalted mixed nuts	100	
Coffee or tea	10	110 Cal
LUNCH		
Turkey frank (2 oz) with mustard & relish	150	
Hot dog bun	130	
Diet soda	0	280 Cal
SNACK		
Yogurt (6 oz, nonfat, any flavor)	90	
Coffee or tea	10	100 Cal
DINNER		
Pasta - Marinara sauce (Day 13 Recipe - page 88)	225	
Large green salad with 1½ Tbsp low-cal dressing	70	
Fresh fruit in season (apple, plum, etc)	70	
Italian or French bread (1 slice)	80	
Glass of red wine (4 oz)	100	
Water with lemon wedge	15	560 Cal
SNACK		
Graham crackers (4 squares)	120	
Coffee or tea	10	130 Cal
		1500 Cal

Day 14 – 1500 Calorie Meal Plan

BREAKFAST	Calories	Totals
Cantaloupe (½ medium)	50	
Oatena cereal mix (Day 14 Recipe - page 89)	310	
Whole-grain toast (1 slice)	65	
Coffee	10	435 Cal
SNACK		
Fresh fruit in season (peach, plum, etc)	70	
Coffee or tea	10	80 Cal
LUNCH		
Grilled Swiss cheese sandwich (2 oz low-fat cheese)	310	
Pickle spear	0	
Gelatin dessert (unsweetened)	10	
Hot or iced tea	10	330 Cal
SNACK		
Handful unsalted mixed nuts	100	
Coffee or tea	10	110 Cal
DINNER		
Frozen chicken dinner (Day 28 Recipe - page 103)	300	
Large green salad with 1½ Tbsp low-cal dressing	70	
Water with lemon wedge	15	385 Cal
SNACK		
Dark chocolate (1 oz)	150	
Coffee or tea	10	160 Cal
		1500 Cal

27

Day 15 – 1500 Calorie Meal Plan

BREAKFAST	Calories	Totals
Fresh or frozen strawberries (1 cup)	50	
French toast (made with 2 slices whole-grain	250	
Light syrup (1 Tbsp)	30	
Coffee	10	340 Cal
SNACK		
Yogurt (6 oz, nonfat, any flavor)	90	
Coffee or tea	10	100 Cal
LUNCH		
Salad (3 oz tuna, 1 tsp Evoo, onions & celery)	175	
Lettuce & tomato wedges	20	
Rye bread (1 slice)	65	
Coffee or tea	10	270 Cal
SNACK		
Handful unsalted mixed nuts	100	
Coffee or tea	10	110 Cal
DINNER		
London broil (Day 15 Recipe - page 90)	320	
Brown rice (½ cup)	100	
Broccoli (1 cup steamed)	50	
Fresh fruit in season (apple, plum, etc)	70	
Hot or iced tea	10	550 Cal
SNACK		
Graham crackers (4 squares)	120	
Coffee or tea	10	130 Cal
		1500 Cal

Day 16 – 1500 Calorie Meal Plan

BREAKFAST	Calories	Totals
Orange juice (½ cup)	50	
Wheat Chex (¾ cup) + ½ cup skim milk + ½ banana	250	
Coffee	10	310 Cal
SNACK		
Fresh fruit in season (peach, plum, etc)	70	
Coffee or tea	10	80 Cal
LUNCH		
Soup (Appendix C - page 113)	100	
Small whole-grain roll	80	
Lettuce and sliced tomato with 1 Tbsp low-cal	45	
Unsweetened apple sauce (½ cup)	45	
Hot or iced tea	10	280 Cal
SNACK		
Popcorn Mini Bag	110	
Coffee or tea	10	120 Cal
DINNER		
Baked red snapper (Day 16 Recipe - page 91)	215	
Wild rice mix	160	
Green beans & tomato	75	
Yogurt (6 oz, nonfat, any flavor)	90	
Water	0	540 Cal
SNACK		
Two small cookies	160	
Coffee or tea	10	170 Cal
		1500 Cal

Day 17 – 1500 Calorie Meal Plan

BREAKFAST	Calories	Totals
Cantaloupe (½ medium)	50	
Fried egg	80	
Turkey bacon (2 slices)	70	
Toasted raisin bread (1 slice)	75	
Coffee	10	285 Cal
SNACK		
Yogurt (6 oz, nonfat, any flavor)	90	
Coffee or tea	10	100 Cal
LUNCH		
Soup (Appendix C - page 113)	170	
Lettuce & tomato sandwich (tsp light mayonnaise)	170	
Gelatin dessert (unsweetened)	10	
Cucumber slices and carrots and celery sticks	15	
Hot or iced tea	10	375 Cal
SNACK		
Handful unsalted mixed nuts	100	100 Cal
DINNER		
Cajun chicken salad (Day 17 Recipe - page 92)	330	
Whole-grain bread (1 slice)	65	
Fresh fruit in season (apple, peach, etc)	70	
Water with lemon wedge	15	480 Cal
SNACK		
Dark chocolate (1 oz)	150	
Coffee or tea	10	160 Cal
		1500 Cal

Day 18 – 1500 Calorie Meal Plan

BREAKFAST	Calories	Totals
Grapefruit (½)	75	
Cheerios (1 cup) + ½ cup skim milk + about 15 raisins	190	
Coffee	10	275 Cal
SNACK		
Fresh fruit in season (peach, plum, etc)	70	
Coffee or tea	10	80 Cal
LUNCH		
Cottage cheese (1 cup low fat)	180	
Large green salad with 1½ Tbsp low-cal dressing	70	
Small whole-grain roll	80	
Hot or iced tea	10	340 Cal
SNACK		
Handful unsalted mixed nuts	100	
Coffee or tea	10	110 Cal
DINNER		
Grilled swordfish (Day 18 Recipe - page 93)	250	
Grilled potatoes	100	
Grilled cherry tomatoes	45	
Spinach (½ cup) steamed w garlic & drizzled Evoo	50	
Whole-grain bread (1 slice)	65	
Water with lemon wedge	15	525 Cal
SNACK		
Two small cookies	160	
Coffee or tea	10	170 Cal
		1500 Cal

31

Day 19 – 1500 Calorie Meal Plan

BREAKFAST	Calories	Totals
Grapefruit (½)	75	
Scrambled egg	80	
Whole grain toast (1 slice)	65	
Coffee	10	230 Cal
SNACK		
Yogurt (6 oz, nonfat, any flavor)	90	
Coffee or tea	10	100 Cal
LUNCH		
Chicken, Bacon Ranch*	270	
Diet soda or water	0	270 Cal
* Hot Pockets (wrap)		
SNACK		
Fresh fruit in season (apple, plum, etc)	70	70 Cal
DINNER		
Eat Out – Chinese food (Day 19 Recipe - page 94)		
Max allowable calories	640	640 Cal
SNACK		
Graham crackers (4 squares)	120	
Skim milk (6 oz)	60	180 Cal
		1500 Cal

Day 20 – 1500 Calorie Meal Plan

BREAKFAST	Calories	Totals
Tomato juice (½ cup)	20	
Shredded Wheat (1 cup) + ½ cup skim milk + ½ banana	260	
Coffee	10	290 Cal
SNACK		
Handful unsalted mixed nuts	100	
Coffee or tea	10	110 Cal
LUNCH		
Left over Chinese food from Day 19	260	
Gelatin dessert (unsweetened)	10	
Hot or iced tea	10	280 Cal
SNACK		
Yogurt (6 oz, nonfat, any flavor)	90	
Coffee or tea	10	100 Cal
DINNER		
Spaghetti alla Puttanesca (Day 20 Recipe - page 95)	345	
Large green salad with 1½ Tbsp low-cal dressing	70	
Italian or French bread (1 slice)	80	
Glass of red wine (4 oz)	100	
Water	0	595 Cal
SNACK		
Graham crackers (4 squares)	120	
Coffee or tea	10	130 Cal
		1505 Cal

Day 21 – 1500 Calorie Meal Plan

BREAKFAST	Calories	Totals
Cantaloupe (½ medium)	50	
Oatmeal (½ cup dry) + ½ cup skim milk + about 15 raisins	220	
Coffee	10	280 Cal
SNACK		
Handful unsalted mixed nuts	100	
Coffee or tea	10	110 Cal
LUNCH		
Turkey breast (2 oz) sandwich	235	
Lettuce, tomato and tsp light mayo	35	
Pickle spear	0	
Fresh fruit in season (apple, plum, etc)	70	
Water	0	340 Cal
SNACK		
Yogurt (6 oz, nonfat, any flavor)	90	90 Cal
DINNER		
Frozen meat dinner (Day 21 Recipe - page 96)	300	
Large green salad with 1½ Tbsp low-cal dressing	70	
Whole-grain bread (1 slice)	65	
Fresh fruit in season (pear, plum, etc)	70	
Water with lemon wedge	15	520 Cal
SNACK		
Dark chocolate (1 oz)	150	
Coffee or tea	10	160 Cal
		1500 Cal

Day 22 – 1500 Calorie Meal Plan

BREAKFAST	Calories	Totals
Fresh or frozen strawberries (½ cup)	25	
French toasted English Muffin (Day 2 Recipe - page 77)	270	
Light syrup (1 Tbsp)	30	
Coffee	10	335 Cal
SNACK		
Fresh fruit in season (pear, plum, etc)	70	
Coffee or tea	10	80 Cal
LUNCH		
Soup (Appendix C - page 113)	130	
BLT sandwich (2 slices turkey bacon, 1 tsp light	235	
Pickle spear	0	
Hot or iced tea	10	375 Cal
SNACK		
Two small cookies	160	
Coffee or tea	10	170 Cal
DINNER		
Shrimp & spinach salad (Day 22 Recipe - page 97)	310	
Whole-grain bread (1 slice)	65	
Large green salad with 1½ Tbsp low-cal dressing	70	
Water	0	445 Cal
SNACK		
Yogurt (6 oz, nonfat, any flavor)	90	
Coffee or tea	10	100 Cal
		1505 Cal

Day 23 – 1500 Calorie Meal Plan

BREAKFAST	Calories	Totals
Cantaloupe (½ medium)	50	
Wheaties (¾ cup) + ½ cup skim milk + ½ banana	190	
Whole-grain toast (1 slice)	65	
Coffee	10	315 Cal
SNACK		
Yogurt (6 oz, nonfat, any flavor)	90	
Coffee or tea	10	100 Cal
LUNCH		
Ham (2 oz) with mustard on 2 slices rye bread	290	
Pickle spear	0	
Small bunch of grapes	65	
Hot or iced tea	10	365 Cal
SNACK		
Handful unsalted mixed nuts	100	
Coffee or tea	10	110 Cal
DINNER		
Beans & greens salad (Day 23 Recipe - page 98)	260	
Whole-grain bread (1 slice)	65	
Baked potato (medium)	100	
Fresh fruit in season (peach, plum, etc)	70	
Water with lemon wedge	15	510 Cal
SNACK		
Graham crackers (3 squares)	90	
Coffee or tea	10	100 Cal
		1500 Cal

Day 24 – 1500 Calorie Meal Plan

BREAKFAST	Calories	Totals
Fresh orange sliced	75	
Soft-boiled egg	80	
Whole-grain toast (2 slices)	130	
Coffee	10	295 Cal
SNACK		
Handful unsalted mixed nuts	100	
Coffee or tea	10	110 Cal
LUNCH		
Salad – 3 oz salmon, 1 tsp Evoo, onions & celery	200	
Lettuce & tomato wedges	20	
Rye bread (1 slice)	65	
Fresh fruit in season (apple, peach, etc)	70	
Coffee or tea	10	365 Cal
SNACK		
Popcorn Mini Bag	110	110 Cal
DINNER		
Chicken breast – broiled (5 oz)	250	
Four bean plus salad - ½ cup (Day 24 Recipe - page 99)	135	
Large green salad with 1½ Tbsp low-cal dressing	70	
Yogurt (6 oz, nonfat, any flavor)	90	
Water	0	545 Cal
SNACK		
Fresh fruit in season (apple, plum, etc)	70	
Coffee or tea	10	80 Cal
		1505 Cal

Day 25 – 1500 Calorie Meal Plan

BREAKFAST	Calories	Totals
Grapefruit (½)	75	
Cheerios (1 cup) + ½ cup skim milk + about 15 raisins	190	
Coffee	10	275 Cal
SNACK		
Fresh fruit in season (apple, peach, etc)	70	
Coffee or tea	10	80 Cal
LUNCH		
Cottage cheese (1 cup low fat)	180	
Large green salad with 1½ Tbsp low-cal dressing	70	
Small whole-grain roll	80	
Water	0	330 Cal
SNACK		
Fiber One Chocolate Fudge Brownie	90	
Coffee or tea	10	100 Cal
DINNER		
Hanger steak (Day 25 Recipe - page 100)	320	
Roasted potatoes (Day 25 Recipe)	120	
Cherry tomatoes (Day 25 Recipe)	20	
Steamed spinach (½ cup)	25	
Whole-grain bread (1 slice)	65	
Water	0	550 Cal
SNACK		
Two small cookies	160	
Coffee or tea	10	170 Cal
		1505 Cal

Day 26 – 1500 Calorie Meal Plan

BREAKFAST	Calories	Totals
Cantaloupe (½ medium)	50	
Fried egg	80	
Toasted whole-grain bread (2 slices)	130	
Coffee	10	270 Cal
SNACK		
Handful unsalted mixed nuts	100	
Coffee or tea	10	110 Cal
LUNCH		
Subway 6" (Ham, Cheese + veggies)	260	
Large green salad with 1½ Tbsp low-cal dressing	70	
Hot or iced tea	10	340 Cal
SNACK		
Fresh fruit in season (apple, plum, etc)	70	
Coffee or tea	10	80 Cal
DINNER		
Grilled scallops (Day 26 Recipe - page 101)	210	
Grilled polenta (Day 26 Recipe.)	125	
For preparation remaining food - see Day 26 Recipe	55	
Yogurt (6 oz, nonfat, any flavor)	90	
Water	0	480 Cal
SNACK		
Graham crackers (5 squares)	150	
Skim milk (6 oz)	70	220 Cal
		1500 Cal

Day 27 – 1500 Calorie Meal Plan

BREAKFAST	Calories	Totals
Cantaloupe (½ medium)	50	
Oatmeal (½ cup dry) + ½ cup skim milk + about 15 raisins	220	
Coffee	10	280 Cal
SNACK		
Fresh fruit in season (apple, plum, etc)	70	
Coffee or tea	10	80 Cal
LUNCH		
Two servings (1 cup) left over Day 24 bean salad	270	
Small whole-grain roll	80	
Lettuce & tomato slices	20	
Hot or iced tea	10	380 Cal
SNACK		
Celery sticks + ¼ cup low-fat cottage cheese & chives	60	
Coffee or tea	10	70 Cal
DINNER		
Fettuccine (Day 27 Recipe - page 102)	290	
Large green salad with 1½ Tbsp low-cal dressing	70	
Italian or French bread (1 slice)	80	
Glass of red wine (4 oz)	100	
Water	0	540 Cal
SNACK		
Dark chocolate (1 oz)	150	150 Cal
		1500 Cal

Day 28 – 1500 Calorie Meal Plan

BREAKFAST	Calories	Totals
Tomato juice (½ cup)	20	
Shredded Wheat (1 cup) + ½ cup skim milk + ½ banana	260	
Coffee	10	290 Cal
SNACK		
Handful unsalted mixed nuts	100	100 Cal
LUNCH		
Roast beef (2 oz) sandwich (whole-grain bread)	295	
Lettuce	0	
Fresh fruit in season (peach, plum, etc)	70	
Hot or iced tea	10	375 Cal
SNACK		
Yogurt (6 oz, nonfat, any flavor)	90	
Coffee or tea	10	100 Cal
DINNER		
Frozen chicken dinner (**Day 28 Recipe** - page 103)	300	
Large green salad with 1½ Tbsp low-cal dressing	70	
Whole-grain bread (1 slice)	65	
Fresh fruit in season (peach, plum, etc)	70	
Water	0	505 Cal
SNACK		
Graham crackers (4 squares)	120	
Coffee or tea	10	130 Cal
		1500 Cal

Day 29 – 1500 Calorie Meal Plan

BREAKFAST	Calories	Totals
Orange juice (½ cup)	50	
Wild blueberry pancakes (Day 10 Recipe - page 85)	190	
Turkey bacon (2 slices)	70	
Light syrup (2 Tbsp)	60	
Coffee	10	380 Cal
SNACK		
Handful unsalted mixed nuts	100	
Coffee or tea	10	110 Cal
LUNCH		
Salad (3 oz tuna, 1 tsp Evoo, onions & celery)	175	
Lettuce & tomato wedges	20	
Rye bread (1 slice)	65	
Fresh fruit in season (pear, peach, etc)	70	
Coffee or tea	10	340 Cal
SNACK		
Fiber One Chocolate Fudge Brownie	90	
Coffee or tea	10	100 Cal
DINNER		
Barbequed shrimp (Day 29 Recipe - page 104)	160	
Corn on the cob (medium)	90	
Steamed broccoli (1 cup equivalent)	60	
Yogurt (6 oz, nonfat, any flavor)	90	
Water	0	400 Cal
SNACK		
Two small cookies	160	
Coffee or tea	10	170 Cal
		1500 Cal

Day 30 – 1500 Calorie Meal Plan

BREAKFAST	Calories	Totals
Fresh orange sliced	75	
Wheat Chex (¾ cup) + ½ cup skim milk + ½ banana	250	
Coffee	10	335 Cal
SNACK		
Fresh fruit in season (peach, plum, etc)	70	
Coffee or tea	10	80 Cal
LUNCH		
Subway 6" (Turkey Breast, Cheese + veggies)	230	
Canned pineapple (½ cup, no-sugar-added juice)	40	
Hot or iced tea	10	280 Cal
SNACK		
Graham crackers (4 squares)	120	
Coffee or tea	10	130 Cal
DINNER		
Cheeseburger (Day 30 Recipe - page 105)	320	
Low-fat American cheese (1 thin slice)	50	
Lettuce and sliced tomato	20	
Whole-grain burger roll	140	
Steamed green beans	25	
Pickle spear	0	
Water	0	555 Cal
SNACK		
Popcorn Mini Bag	110	
Coffee or tea	10	120 Cal
		1500 Cal

1800-Calorie
Daily Menus

Day 1 – 1800 Calorie Meal Plan

BREAKFAST	Calories	Totals
Orange juice (½ cup)	50	
Wheaties (¾ cup) + ½ cup skim milk + ½ banana	190	
Whole-grain toast (2 slices) (See page 8)	130	
Coffee (See Notes - page 11)	10	380 Cal
SNACK		
Fresh fruit in season (apple, peach, etc)	70	
Coffee or tea	10	80 Cal
LUNCH		
Soup (Appendix C - page 113)	110	
Turkey breast (3 oz) on rye bread sandwich	260	
Pickle spear	0	
Lettuce & tomato slices	20	
Hot or iced tea	10	400 Cal
SNACK		
Two small cookies (oatmeal, etc - check calories!)	160	
Skim milk (6 oz)	60	220 Cal
DINNER		
Baked Herb-Crusted Cod (Day 1 Recipe - page 76)	230	
For preparation remaining food - see Day 1 Recipe	120	
Baked potato (medium)	100	
Large green salad with 1½ Tbsp low-cal dressing	70	
Whole grain bread (1 slice)	65	
Water with lemon wedge	15	600 Cal
SNACK		
Popcorn Mini Bag*	110	
Coffee or tea	10	120 Cal
* Such as Orville Redenbacher's Smart Pop		1800 Cal

45

Day 2 – 1800 Calorie Meal Plan

BREAKFAST	Calories	Totals
Fresh or frozen strawberries (½ cup)	25	
French toasted English muffins (Day 2 Recipe - page 77)	360	
Light syrup (1 Tbsp)	30	
Coffee	10	425 Cal
SNACK		
Yogurt (6 oz, nonfat, any flavor)	90	
Coffee or tea	10	100 Cal
LUNCH		
Salad (3 oz tuna, 1 tsp Evoo, onions & celery)	175	
Lettuce & tomato wedges	20	
Rye bread (1 slice)	65	
Fresh fruit in season (apple, plum, etc)	70	
Coffee or tea	10	380 Cal
SNACK		
Handful unsalted mixed nuts	100	
Coffee or tea	10	110 Cal
DINNER		
Broiled veal chop (6 oz lean)	300	
Corn on the cob (1 medium ear)	100	
Broccoli (1 cup steamed & drizzled with 1 tsp	95	
Large green salad with 1½ Tbsp low-cal dressing	70	
Hot or iced tea	10	575 Cal
SNACK		
Graham crackers (4 squares)	120	
Skim milk (8 oz)	90	210 Cal
		1800 Cal

Day 3 – 1800 Calorie Meal Plan

BREAKFAST	Calories	Totals
Grapefruit (½)	75	
Scrambled eggs (2 eggs - see Notes - page 11)	160	
Turkey bacon (2 slices)	70	
Whole-grain toast (2 slices)	130	
Coffee	10	445 Cal
SNACK		
Yogurt (6 oz, nonfat, any flavor)	90	
Coffee or tea	10	100 Cal
LUNCH		
Ham (3 oz) w mustard - 2 slices whole-grain bread	370	
Lettuce & tomato slices	20	
Small bunch grapes	65	
Water	0	455 Cal
SNACK		
Handful unsalted mixed nuts	100	100 Cal
DINNER		
Chicken w Peppers & Onions (Day 3 Recipe - page 78)	250	
For preparation remaining food - see Day 3 Recipe	125	
Large green salad with 1½ Tbsp low-cal dressing	70	
Whole-grain bread (1 slice)	65	
Fresh fruit in season (pear, plum, etc)	70	
Water	0	580 Cal
SNACK		
Popcorn Mini Bag	110	
Coffee or tea	10	120 Cal
		1800 Cal

Day 4 – 1800 Calorie Meal Plan

BREAKFAST	Calories	Totals
Grapefruit (½)	75	
Cheerios (1 cup) + ½ cup skim milk + about 15 raisins*	190	
Whole-grain toast (1 slice)	65	
Coffee	10	340 Cal
SNACK		
Fresh fruit in season (apple, plum, etc)	70	
Coffee or tea	10	80 Cal
LUNCH		
Subway 6" (Ham, Cheese + veggies)*	260	
Canned pineapple (1 cup, no-sugar-added juice)	80	
Water with lemon wedge	10	350 Cal
* On 6" half wheat roll.		
SNACK		
Handful unsalted mixed nuts	100	
Coffee or tea	10	110 Cal
DINNER		
Meat Loaf [1½ servings] (Day 4 Recipe - page 79)	435	
For preparation remaining food - see Day 4 Recipe	185	
Romaine lettuce, tomato slices & 1 Tbsp low-cal	45	
Whole-grain bread (1 slice)	65	
Gelatin dessert (unsweetened)	10	
Hot or iced tea	10	750 Cal
SNACK		
Two small cookies	160	
Coffee or tea	10	170 Cal
* See Notes re substituting blueberries for raisins.		1800 Cal

Day 5 – 1800 Calorie Meal Plan

BREAKFAST	Calories	Totals
Cantaloupe (½ medium)	50	
Fried eggs (2 eggs)	160	
Turkey bacon (2 slices)	70	
Toasted raisin bread (2 slices)	150	
Coffee	10	440 Cal
SNACK		
Yogurt (6 oz, nonfat, any flavor)	90	
Coffee or tea	10	100 Cal
LUNCH		
Soup (Appendix C - page 113)	190	
Small whole-grain roll	80	
Lettuce and sliced tomato with 1 Tbsp low-cal	45	
Canned pineapple (½ cup, no-sugar-added juice)	40	
Hot or iced tea	10	365 Cal
SNACK		
Dark chocolate (1 oz)	150	
Coffee or tea	10	160 Cal
DINNER		
Frozen fish dinner (Day 5 Recipe - page 80)	340	
Large green salad with 1½ Tbsp low-cal dressing	70	
Steamed cauliflower (1 cup)	25	
Whole-grain bread (1 slice)	65	
Fresh fruit in season (apple, peach, etc)	70	
Hot or iced tea	10	580 Cal
SNACK		
Skinny Cow Ice Cream Sandwich	140	
Coffee or tea	10	150 Cal
		1805 Cal

Day 6 – 1800 Calorie Meal Plan

BREAKFAST	Calories	Totals
Tomato juice (½ cup)	20	
Shredded Wheat (1 cup) + ½ cup skim milk + ½ banana	265	
Whole-grain toast (2 slices)	130	
Coffee	10	425 Cal
SNACK		
Handful unsalted mixed nuts	100	
Coffee or tea	10	110 Cal
LUNCH		
Leftover meat loaf (Day 4 serving size) - ketchup	290	
Small whole-grain roll	80	
Lettuce	0	
Fresh or frozen berries (½ cup)	50	
Hot or iced tea	10	430 Cal
SNACK		
Yogurt (6 oz, nonfat, any flavor)	90	
Coffee or tea	10	100 Cal
DINNER		
Pizza (Day 6 Recipe - page 81)	350	
Large green salad with 1½ Tbsp low-cal dressing	70	
Glass of red wine (4 oz)	100	
Fresh fruit in season (apple, peach, etc)	70	
Water with lemon wedge	15	605 Cal
SNACK		
Graham Crackers (4 squares)	120	
Coffee or tea	10	130 Cal
		1800 Cal

Day 7 – 1800 Calorie Meal Plan

BREAKFAST	Calories	Totals
Cantaloupe (½ medium)	50	
Oatmeal (½ cup dry) + ½ cup skim milk + about 15 raisins	220	
Whole-grain toast (2 slices)	130	
Coffee	10	410 Cal
SNACK		
Fresh fruit in season (apple, plum, etc)	70	
Coffee or tea	10	80 Cal
LUNCH		
Soup (Appendix C - page 113)	90	
Grilled cheese sandwich (2 slices 2% American	230	
Lettuce and sliced tomato	20	
Pickle spear	0	
Diet soda or water	0	340 Cal
SNACK		
Popcorn Mini Bag	110	
Coffee or tea	10	120 Cal
DINNER		
Eat Out – Chicken dinner (Day 7 Recipe - page 82)		
Max allowable calories	630	630 Cal
SNACK		
Graham crackers (5 squares)	150	
Skim milk (6 oz)	70	220 Cal
		1800 Cal

Day 8 – 1800 Calorie Meal Plan

BREAKFAST	Calories	Totals
Cantaloupe (½ medium)	50	
Wheaties (¾ cup) + ½ cup skim milk + ½ banana	190	
Whole-grain toast (2 slices)	130	
Coffee	10	380 Cal
SNACK		
Fresh fruit in season (apple, plum, etc)	70	70 Cal
LUNCH		
Soup (Appendix C - page 113)	140	
Turkey (2 oz) sandwich	230	
Lettuce & tomato slices	20	
Yogurt (6 oz, nonfat, any flavor)	90	
Hot or iced tea	10	490 Cal
SNACK		
Two small cookies	160	
Coffee or tea	10	170 Cal
DINNER		
Baked salmon with salsa (Day 8 Recipe - page 83)	215	
Summer squash, zucchini and tomatoes	60	
Brown rice (¾ cup)	150	
Large green salad with 1½ Tbsp low-cal dressing	70	
Fresh fruit in season (apple, peach, etc)	70	
Water	0	565 Cal
SNACK		
Popcorn Mini Bag	110	
Coffee or tea	10	120 Cal
		1800 Cal

Day 9 – 1800 Calorie Meal Plan

BREAKFAST	Calories	Totals
Orange juice (½ cup)	50	
Fried eggs (2 eggs)	160	
Whole-grain toast (2 slices)	130	
Turkey bacon (2 slices)	70	
Coffee	10	420 Cal
SNACK		
Yogurt (6 oz, nonfat) & ½ cup fresh or frozen berries	140	
Coffee or tea	10	150 Cal
LUNCH		
Tuna salad (4 oz tuna, 1 tsp Evoo, onions & celery)	215	
Lettuce & tomato wedges + rye bread (1 slice)	85	
Fresh fruit in season – (apple, peach, etc)	70	
Whole-grain bread (1 slice)	65	
Hot or iced tea	10	445 Cal
SNACK		
Handful unsalted mixed nuts	100	
Coffee or tea	10	110 Cal
DINNER		
Veggie burger – (1 patty) (Day 9 Recipe - page 84)	100	
Low-fat cheddar cheese (2 thin slices)	100	
Beets (3 small) + seeded burger roll	185	
Large green salad with 1½ Tbsp low-cal dressing	70	
Fresh fruit in season (peach, plum, etc)	70	
Water with lemon wedge	15	540 Cal
SNACK		
Graham crackers (4 squares)	120	
Coffee or tea	10	130 Cal
		1795 Cal

Day 10 – 1800 Calorie Meal Plan

BREAKFAST	Calories	Totals
Orange juice (½ cup)	50	
Wild blueberry pancakes (Day 10 Recipe - page 85)	190	
Turkey bacon (2 slices)	70	
Light syrup (1½ Tbsp)	45	
Coffee	10	365 Cal
SNACK		
Handful unsalted mixed nuts	100	100 Cal
LUNCH		
Peanut butter (2 Tbsp) + 2 slices whole-grain bread	330	
Skim milk (8 oz)	90	
Carrot sticks + ¼ cup low-fat cottage cheese & chives	60	
Fresh fruit in season (apple, plum, etc)	70	550 Cal
SNACK		
Fiber One Chocolate Fudge Brownie	90	
Coffee or tea	10	100 Cal
DINNER		
Soup (Appendix C - page 113)	100	
Broiled pork chop (about ½" thick, trimmed of fat)	260	
Green peas (½ cup)	55	
Tomato & cucumber salad with 1½ Tbsp low-cal	70	
Whole-grain bread (1 slice)	65	
Water with lemon wedge	15	565 Cal
SNACK		
Popcorn Mini Bag	110	
Coffee or tea	10	120 Cal
		1800 Cal

Day 11 – 1800 Calorie Meal Plan

BREAKFAST	Calories	Totals
Fresh sliced orange	75	
Cheerios (1 cup) + ½ cup skim milk + about 15 raisins	190	
Whole-grain toast (2 slices)	130	
Coffee	10	405 Cal
SNACK		
Fresh fruit in season (peach, plum, etc)	70	
Coffee or tea	10	80 Cal
LUNCH		
Cottage cheese (1 cup low fat)	180	
Large green salad with 1½ Tbsp low-cal dressing	70	
Small whole-grain roll	80	
Hot or iced tea	10	340 Cal
SNACK		
"Large" handful unsalted mixed nuts	150	150 Cal
DINNER		
Grilled chicken sausage (3 links about 2½ oz per link)	270	
Artichoke-bean salad (Day 11 Recipe - page 86)	190	
Green beans - steamed	25	
Glass of wine (4 oz)	100	
Hot or iced tea	10	595 Cal
SNACK		
Two small cookies	160	
Skim milk (6 oz)	70	220 Cal
		1800 Cal

Day 12 – 1800 Calorie Meal Plan

BREAKFAST	Calories	Totals
Grapefruit (½)	75	
Scrambled eggs (2 eggs)	160	
Turkey bacon (2 slices)	70	
Whole-grain toast (2 slices)	130	
Coffee	10	445 Cal
SNACK		
Yogurt (6 oz, nonfat, any flavor)	90	
Coffee or tea	10	100 Cal
LUNCH		
Soup (Appendix C - page 113)	150	
Open face ham sandwich (2 oz ham)	225	
Tomato slices + ¼ cup chopped fresh basil & 1 tsp Evoo	60	
Gelatin dessert (unsweetened)	10	
Hot or iced tea	10	455 Cal
SNACK		
Fresh fruit in season (pear, plum, etc)	70	
Coffee or tea	10	80 Cal
DINNER		
Eat Out – Fish dinner (Day 12 Recipe - page 87)		
Max allowable calories	595	595 Cal
SNACK		
Graham crackers (4 squares)	120	
Coffee or tea	10	130 Cal
		1805 Cal

Day 13 – 1800 Calorie Meal Plan

BREAKFAST	Calories	Totals
Orange juice (½ cup)	50	
Shredded Wheat (1 cup) + ½ cup skim milk + ½ banana	260	
Whole-grain toast (2 slices)	130	
Coffee	10	450 Cal
SNACK		
Handful unsalted mixed nuts	100	
Coffee or tea	10	110 Cal
LUNCH		
Turkey frank (2 oz) with mustard & relish	150	
Hot-dog bun	130	
Yogurt (6 oz, nonfat) & ½ cup fresh or frozen	140	
Hot or iced tea	10	430 Cal
SNACK		
Graham crackers (4 squares)	120	
Coffee or tea	10	130 Cal
DINNER		
Pasta - Marinara sauce (Day 13 Recipe - page 88)	225	
Large green salad with 1½ Tbsp low-cal dressing	70	
Italian or French bread (1 slice)	80	
Glass of red wine (4 oz)	100	
Water with lemon wedge	15	
Fresh fruit in season (apple, plum, etc)	70	560 Cal
SNACK		
Popcorn Mini Bag	110	
Coffee or tea	10	120 Cal
		1800 Cal

Day 14 – 1800 Calorie Meal Plan

BREAKFAST	Calories	Totals
Cantaloupe (½ medium)	50	
Oatena cereal mix (Day 14 Recipe - page 90)	310	
Whole-grain toast (2 slices)	130	
Coffee	10	500 Cal
SNACK		
Fresh fruit in season (pear, plum, etc)	70	
Coffee or tea	10	80 Cal
LUNCH		
Grilled Swiss cheese sandwich (2 oz low-fat cheese)	280	
Turkey bacon (2 slices for sandwich)	70	
Pickle spear	0	
Gelatin dessert (unsweetened)	10	
Water with lemon wedge	15	375 Cal
SNACK		
Handful unsalted mixed nuts	100	
Coffee or tea	10	110 Cal
DINNER		
Frozen chicken dinner (Day 28 Recipe - page 103)	300	
Large green salad with 1½ Tbsp low-cal dressing	70	
Whole-grain bread (1 slice)	65	
Yogurt (6 oz, nonfat) & ½ cup fresh or frozen berries	140	
Water	0	575 Cal
SNACK		
Dark chocolate (1 oz)	150	
Coffee or tea	10	160 Cal
		1800 Cal

Day 15 – 1800 Calorie Meal Plan

BREAKFAST	Calories	Totals
Fresh or frozen strawberries (1 cup)	50	
French toast (3 slices whole-grain bread)	250	
Light syrup (2 Tbsp)	60	
Coffee	10	495 Cal
SNACK		
Yogurt (6 oz, nonfat, any flavor)	90	
Coffee or tea	10	100 Cal
LUNCH		
Salad (4 oz tuna, 1 tsp Evoo, onions & celery)	215	
Lettuce & tomato wedges	20	
Rye bread (1 slice)	65	
Gelatin dessert (unsweetened)	10	
Coffee or tea	10	320 Cal
SNACK		
Handful unsalted mixed nuts	100	
Coffee or tea	10	110 Cal
DINNER		
London broil (Day 15 Recipe - page 90)	320	
Brown rice (½ cup)	100	
Broccoli (1 cup steamed)	50	
Fresh fruit in season (apple, peach, etc)	70	
Water with lemon wedge	15	555 Cal
SNACK		
Graham crackers (5 squares)	150	
Skim milk (6 oz)	70	220 Cal
		1800 Cal

Day 16 – 1800 Calorie Meal Plan

BREAKFAST	Calories	Totals
Orange juice (½ cup)	50	
Wheat Chex (¾ cup) + ½ cup skim milk + ½ banana	250	
Whole-grain toast (2 slices)	130	
Coffee	10	440 Cal
## SNACK		
Fresh fruit in season (apple, plum, etc)	70	
Coffee or tea	10	80 Cal
## LUNCH		
Chicken, Broccoli & Cheese*	270	
Lettuce and sliced tomato with 1 Tbsp low-cal	45	
Unsweetened apple sauce (½ cup)	45	
Diet soda or water	0	360 Cal
* Hot Pockets Wrap		
## SNACK		
Kashi Crunchy Granola Bar	180	
Coffee or tea	10	190 Cal
## DINNER		
Baked red snapper (Day 16 Recipe - page 91)	215	
Wild rice mix (¾ cup - cooked)	160	
Green beans & tomato (Day 16 Recipe)	75	
Whole-grain bread (1 slice)	65	
Fresh fruit in season (apple, plum, etc)	70	
Water	0	585 Cal
## SNACK		
Skinny Cow Ice Cream Sandwich	140	
Coffee or tea	10	150 Cal
		1805 Cal

Day 17 – 1800 Calorie Meal Plan

BREAKFAST	Calories	Totals
Cantaloupe (½ medium)	50	
Fried eggs (2 eggs)	160	
Turkey bacon (2 slices)	70	
Toasted raisin bread (2 slices)	150	
Coffee	10	440 Cal
SNACK		
Yogurt (6 oz, nonfat) & ½ cup fresh or frozen berries	140	
Coffee or tea	10	150 Cal
LUNCH		
Soup (Appendix C - page 113)	180	
Lettuce & tomato sandwich (tsp light mayonnaise)	170	
Cucumber slices, carrots & celery sticks	15	
Gelatin dessert (unsweetened)	10	
Hot or iced tea	10	385 Cal
SNACK		
Handful unsalted mixed nuts	100	
Coffee or tea	10	110 Cal
DINNER		
Cajun chicken salad (Day 17 Recipe - page 92)	330	
Whole-grain bread (1 slice)	65	
Fresh fruit in season (apple, peach, etc)	70	
Water with lemon wedge	15	495 Cal
SNACK		
Graham crackers (5 squares)	150	
Skim milk (6 oz)	70	220 Cal
		1800 Cal

Day 18 – 1800 Calorie Meal Plan

BREAKFAST	Calories	Totals
Grapefruit (½)	75	
Cheerios (1 cup) + ½ cup skim milk + about 15 raisins	190	
Whole-grain toast (2 slices)	130	
Coffee	10	405 Cal
SNACK		
Handful unsalted mixed nuts	100	
Coffee or tea	10	110 Cal
LUNCH		
Cottage cheese (1 cup low fat)	180	
Large tossed green salad with 1½ Tbsp low-cal	70	
Small whole-grain roll	80	
Hot or iced tea	10	340 Cal
SNACK		
Yogurt (6 oz, nonfat, any flavor)	90	
Coffee or tea	10	100 Cal
DINNER		
Grilled swordfish (Day 18 Recipe - page 93)	250	
Grilled potatoes	100	
Grilled cherry tomatoes	45	
Spinach (½ cup) steamed with garlic & drizzled	50	
Whole-grain bread (1 slice)	65	
Fresh fruit in season (apple, plum, etc)	70	
Water with lemon wedge	15	595 Cal
SNACK		
Two small cookies	160	
Skim milk (8 oz)*	90	250 Cal
* Instead you could have 8 oz non-fat yogurt.		1800 Cal

Day 19 – 1800 Calorie Meal Plan

BREAKFAST	Calories	Totals
Grapefruit (½)	75	
Scrambled eggs (2 eggs)	160	
Whole-grain toast (2 slices)	130	
Turkey bacon (1 slice)	35	
Coffee	10	410 Cal
SNACK		
Yogurt (6 oz, nonfat, any flavor)	90	
Coffee or tea	10	100 Cal
LUNCH		
Soup (Appendix C - page 113)	130	
Turkey sandwich (2 oz turkey breast)	230	
Lettuce & tomato slices	20	
Hot or iced tea	10	390 Cal
SNACK		
Fresh fruit in season (pear, plum, etc)	70	
Coffee or tea	10	80 Cal
DINNER		
Eat Out – Chinese food (Day 19 Recipe - page 94)		
Max allowable calories	640	640 Cal
SNACK		
Graham crackers (4 squares)	120	
Skim milk (6 oz)*	60	180 Cal
* Instead you could have 6 oz non-fat yogurt.		1800 Cal

Day 20 – 1800 Calorie Meal Plan

BREAKFAST	Calories	Totals
Tomato juice (½ cup)	20	
Shredded Wheat (1 cup) + ½ cup skim milk + ½ banana	260	
Raisin-bread toast (2 slices)	150	
Coffee	10	440 Cal
SNACK		
Handful unsalted mixed nuts	100	
Coffee or tea	10	110 Cal
LUNCH		
Left over Chinese food from Day 19	260	
Fresh fruit in season (peach, plum, etc)	70	
Gelatin dessert (unsweetened)	10	
Hot or iced tea	10	350 Cal
SNACK		
Yogurt (6 oz, nonfat) & ½ cup fresh or frozen berries	140	
Coffee or tea	10	150 Cal
DINNER		
Spaghetti alla Puttanesca (Day 20 Recipe - page 95)	345	
Large green salad with 1½ Tbsp low-cal dressing	70	
Italian or French bread (1 slice)	80	
Glass of red wine (4 oz)	100	
Water with lemon wedge	15	610 Cal
SNACK		
Popcorn Mini Bag	110	
Coffee or tea	10	120 Cal
		1780 Cal

Day 21 – 1800 Calorie Meal Plan

BREAKFAST	Calories	Totals
Cantaloupe (½ medium)	50	
Oatmeal (½ cup dry) + ½ cup skim milk + about 15 raisins	220	
Whole-grain toast (2 slices)	130	
Coffee	10	410 Cal
SNACK		
Handful unsalted mixed nuts	100	
Coffee or tea	10	110 Cal
LUNCH		
Turkey breast (3 oz) sandwich	285	
Lettuce, tomato and tsp light mayo	35	
Pickle spear	0	
Banana (medium)	100	
Water with lemon wedge	15	435 Cal
SNACK		
Yogurt (6 oz, nonfat) & ½ cup fresh or frozen berries	140	
Coffee or tea	10	150 Cal
DINNER		
Frozen meat dinner (Day 21 Recipe - page 96)	300	
Large tossed green salad with 1½ Tbsp low-cal	70	
Whole-grain bread (1 slice)	65	
Fresh fruit in season (pear, plum, etc)	70	
Gelatin dessert (unsweetened)	10	
Water with lemon wedge	15	530 Cal
SNACK		
Dark chocolate (1 oz)	150	
Coffee or tea	10	160 Cal
		1795 Cal

Day 22 – 1800 Calorie Meal Plan

BREAKFAST	Calories	Totals
Fresh or frozen strawberries (1 cup)	25	
French toasted English muffins (Day 2 Recipe - page 77)	360	
Light syrup (1 Tbsp)	30	
Coffee	10	425 Cal
SNACK		
Fresh fruit in season (apple, peach, etc)	70	
Coffee or tea	10	80 Cal
LUNCH		
Soup (Appendix C - page 113)	140	
BLT sandwich (2 slices turkey bacon, 1 tsp light	235	
Yogurt (6 oz, nonfat, any flavor)	90	
Hot or iced tea	10	475 Cal
SNACK		
Popcorn Mini Bag	110	
Coffee or tea	10	120 Cal
DINNER		
Shrimp & spinach salad (Day 22 Recipe - page 97)	310	
Whole-grain bread (1 slice)	65	
Fresh fruit in season (apple, plum, etc)	70	
Water with lemon wedge	15	460 Cal
SNACK		
Two small cookies	160	
Skim milk (6 oz)*	70	230 Cal
* Instead you could have 6 oz non-fat yogurt.		1790 Cal

Day 23 – 1800 Calorie Meal Plan

BREAKFAST	Calories	Totals
Cantaloupe (½ medium)	50	
Wheaties (¾ cup) + ½ cup skim milk + ½ banana	190	
Whole-grain toast (2 slices)	130	
Coffee	10	380 Cal
SNACK		
Yogurt (6 oz, nonfat) & ½ cup fresh or frozen berries	140	
Coffee or tea	10	150 Cal
LUNCH		
Ham (3 oz) with mustard on 2 slices rye bread	370	
Pickle spear	0	
Small bunch of grapes	65	
Water with lemon wedge	15	450 Cal
SNACK		
Handful unsalted mixed nuts	100	
Coffee or tea	10	110 Cal
DINNER		
Beans & greens salad (Day 23 Recipe - page 98)	260	
Baked potato (medium)	100	
Whole-grain bread (1 slice)	65	
Fresh fruit in season (apple, plum, etc)	70	
Water with lemon wedge	15	510 Cal
SNACK		
Graham crackers (4 squares)*	120	
Skim milk (6 oz)*	70	190 Cal
* Instead you could have 6 oz non-fat yogurt.		1790 Cal

Day 24 – 1800 Calorie Meal Plan

BREAKFAST	Calories	Totals
Fresh orange sliced	75	
Soft-boiled (or poached) eggs (2 eggs)	160	
Whole-grain toast (2 slices)	130	
Coffee	10	375 Cal
SNACK		
Yogurt (6 oz, nonfat) & ½ cup fresh or frozen berries	140	
Coffee or tea	10	150 Cal
LUNCH		
Salad – 3 oz salmon, 1 tsp Evoo, onions & celery	200	
Lettuce & tomato wedges	20	
Rye bread (1 slice)	65	
Fresh fruit in season (apple, peach, etc)	70	
Hot or iced tea	10	365 Cal
SNACK		
Fiber One Chocolate Fudge Brownie	90	
Coffee or tea	10	100 Cal
DINNER		
Soup (Appendix C - page 113)	110	
Chicken breast – broiled (6 oz)	300	
Four bean plus salad - ½ cup (Day 24 Recipe -page 99)	135	
Large green salad with 1½ Tbsp low-cal dressing	70	
Gelatin dessert (unsweetened)	10	
Water with lemon wedge	15	640 Cal
SNACK		
100-Calorie Pack Cookies*	100	
Skim milk (6 oz)	60	160 Cal
* Such as Nabisco Oreos/Chips Ahoy/etc.		1790 Cal

Day 25 – 1800 Calorie Meal Plan

BREAKFAST	Calories	Totals
Grapefruit (½)	75	
Cheerios (1 cup) + ½ cup skim milk + about 15 raisins	190	
Whole-grain toast (2 slices)	130	
Coffee	10	405 Cal
SNACK		
Popcorn Mini Bag	110	
Coffee or tea	10	120 Cal
LUNCH		
Cottage cheese (1 cup low fat)	180	
Large green salad with 1½ Tbsp low-cal dressing	70	
Small whole-grain roll	80	
Hot or iced tea	10	340 Cal
SNACK		
Fiber One Chocolate Fudge Brownie	90	
Coffee or tea	10	100 Cal
DINNER		
Hanger steak (Day 25 Recipe - page 100)	320	
Roasted potatoes (Day 25 Recipe)	120	
Cherry tomatoes (Day 25 Recipe)	20	
Steamed spinach (½ cup)	25	
Whole-grain bread (1 slice)	65	
Fresh fruit in season (pear, plum, etc)	70	
Water with lemon wedge	15	635 Cal
SNACK		
Kashi Crunchy Granola Bar	180	
Coffee or tea	10	190 Cal
		1790 Cal

Day 26 – 1800 Calorie Meal Plan

BREAKFAST	Calories	Totals
Cantaloupe (½ medium)	50	
Fried eggs (2 eggs)	160	
Turkey bacon (2 slices)	70	
Toasted whole-grain bread (2 slices)	130	
Coffee	10	420 Cal
SNACK		
Yogurt (6 oz, nonfat) & ½ cup fresh or frozen berries	140	
Coffee or tea	10	150 Cal
LUNCH		
Soup (Appendix C - page 113)*	300	
Small whole-grain roll	80	
Lettuce & tomato slices	20	
Hot or iced tea	10	410 Cal
* Enjoy 2 servings of a 150 Cal soup.		
SNACK		
Kashi Chewy Granola Bar	140	
Coffee or tea	10	150 Cal
DINNER		
Grilled scallops (Day 26 Recipe - page 101)	210	
Grilled polenta (Day 26 Recipe)	125	
Grilled mushroom steamed green beans, onions, asparagus	55	
Fresh fruit in season (apple, plum, etc)	70	
Water with lemon wedge	15	475 Cal
SNACK		
Graham crackers (4 squares)	120	
Skim milk (6 oz)	70	190 Cal
		1795 Cal

Day 27 – 1800 Calorie Meal Plan

BREAKFAST	Calories	Totals
Cantaloupe (½ medium)	50	
Oatmeal (½ cup dry) + ½ cup skim milk + about 15 raisins	220	
Whole-grain toast (2 slices)	130	
Coffee	10	410 Cal
SNACK		
Fresh fruit in season (apple, plum, etc)	70	
Coffee or tea	10	80 Cal
LUNCH		
Two servings (1 cup) left over Day 24 bean salad	270	
Small whole-grain roll	80	
Lettuce & tomato slices	20	
Yogurt (6 oz, nonfat, any flavor)	90	
Hot or iced tea	10	470 Cal
SNACK		
Handful unsalted mixed nuts	100	
Coffee or tea	10	110 Cal
DINNER		
Fettuccine (Day 27 Recipe - page 102)	290	
Large green salad with 1½ Tbsp low-cal dressing	70	
Italian or French bread (1 slice)	80	
Glass red wine (4 oz)	100	
Water with lemon wedge	15	555 Cal
SNACK		
Dark chocolate (1 oz)	150	
Coffee or tea	10	160 Cal
		1785 Cal

Day 28 – 1800 Calorie Meal Plan

BREAKFAST	Calories	Totals
Tomato juice (½ cup)	20	
Shredded Wheat (1 cup) + ½ cup skim milk + ½ banana	260	
Raisin-bread toast (2 slices)	150	
Coffee	10	440 Cal
SNACK		
"Large" handful unsalted mixed nuts	150	
Coffee or tea	10	160 Cal
LUNCH		
Roast beef (3 oz) sandwich (whole-grain bread)	370	
Lettuce and tomato slices	20	
Fresh fruit in season (pear, plum, etc)	70	
Hot or iced tea	10	470 Cal
SNACK		
Fiber One Chocolate Fudge Brownie	90	
Coffee or tea	10	100 Cal
DINNER		
Frozen chicken dinner (Day 28 Recipe - page 103)	300	
Large green salad with 1½ Tbsp low-cal dressing	70	
Whole-grain bread (1 slice)	65	
Water with lemon wedge	15	450 Cal
SNACK		
Graham crackers (4 squares)	120	
Skim milk (6 oz)	60	180 Cal
		1800 Cal

Day 29 – 1800 Calorie Meal Plan

BREAKFAST	Calories	Totals
Orange juice (½ cup)	50	
Wild blueberry pancakes (Day 10 Recipe - page 85)	190	
Turkey bacon (2 slices)	70	
Light syrup (1½ Tbsp)	45	
Coffee	10	365 Cal
SNACK		
Yogurt (6 oz, nonfat) & ½ cup fresh or frozen berries	140	
Coffee or tea	10	150 Cal
LUNCH		
Salad (4 oz tuna, 1 tsp Evoo, onions & celery)	215	
Lettuce & tomato wedges	20	
Rye bread (1 slice)	65	
Fresh fruit in season (pear, peach, etc)	70	
Coffee or tea	10	380 Cal
SNACK		
"Large" handful unsalted mixed nuts	150	
Coffee or tea	10	160 Cal
DINNER		
Soup (Appendix C - page 113)	130	
Barbequed shrimp (Day 29 Recipe - page 104)	160	
Corn on the cob (medium)	100	
Steamed broccoli (1 cup) + Whole-grain bread (1 slice)	50	
Water with lemon wedge	15	520 Cal
SNACK		
Two small cookies	160	
Skim milk (6 oz)	70	230 Cal
		1805 Cal

Day 30 – 1800 Calorie Meal Plan

BREAKFAST	Calories	Totals
Orange juice (½ cup)	50	
Wheat Chex (¾ cup) + ½ cup skim milk + ½ banana	250	
Whole-grain toast (2 slices)	130	
Coffee	10	440 Cal
SNACK		
Fresh fruit in season (apple, peach, etc)	70	
Coffee or tea	10	80 Cal
LUNCH		
Soup (Appendix C - page 113)	140	
Small whole-grain roll	80	
Raw zucchini slices, celery & carrot sticks	20	
Canned pineapple (½ cup, no-sugar-added juice)	40	
Hot or iced tea	10	290 Cal
SNACK		
Graham crackers (4 squares)	120	
Skim milk (6 oz)	60	180 Cal
DINNER		
Cheeseburger (Day 30 Recipe - page 105)	320	
Low-fat American cheese (2 thin slices)	100	
Lettuce and sliced tomato & steamed green beans	45	
Whole-grain burger roll	140	
Large salad with 1½ Tbsp low-cal dressing	70	
Water with lemon wedge	15	690 Cal
SNACK		
Popcorn Mini Bag	110	
Coffee or tea	10	120 Cal
		1800 Cal

Recipes & Diet Tips

Day 1 Recipe
Baked Herb-Crusted Cod

4 cod fish fillets (4 to 5 ounces each)
2 tablespoons flour
2 tablespoons cornmeal
2 tablespoons minced fresh herbs
2 teaspoons lemon juice

Sprinkle cod with lemon juice. Mix flour, cornmeal and herbs and dust the cod with the cornmeal-herb mixture. Bake in oven at 375 °F for 10 minutes. Add salt and black pepper to taste.
Serves 4. One serving is about 230 Calories (for cod only).

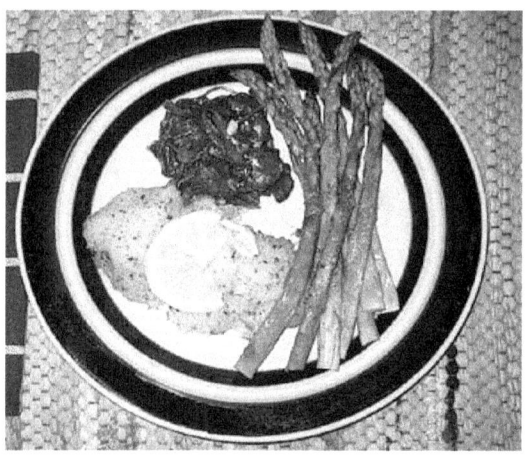

Diet Tip of the Day:. A **reducing diet is best supervised by a physician**. This is especially true when a great deal of weight needs to be lost, or if you have an ailment or a history of medical problems.

Day 2 Recipe
<u>French-Toasted English Muffin</u>

6 whole wheat English muffins (light)

4 eggs

2 cups skim milk

2 teaspoons (tsp) vanilla

Dash of cinnamon

In a medium bowl, beat together eggs and skim milk. Add vanilla and cinnamon. Separate English muffins into halves and saturate slices in egg mixture. In a non-stick skillet coated with cooking spray, cook muffins until both sides are golden brown. Dust lightly with confectionary sugar. Serve hot or keep in an oven or warmer at 200 °F until ready to plate. **Serves 4**. Three English muffin slices (1½ muffins) per serving. Serving is 270 Calories.

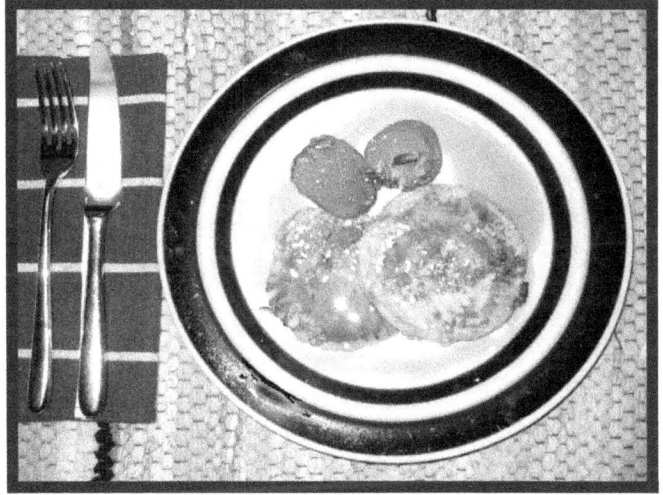

Diet Tip of the Day: **"Eat Slowly"** This is especially vital when you are trying to lose weight. If you are someone who eats fast, who finishes before everyone else at the table, you are not giving yourself a chance to feel full. While everyone else is still eating, you either sit there and pick, or you have seconds, taking in extra calories you could avoid if you would just slow down.

Day 3 Recipe
<u>Chicken with Peppers & Onions</u>
4 boneless & skinless chicken breasts (about 5 oz each)

Coat the chicken breasts in a bottled barbeque sauce. Prepare medium-hot fire on well-oiled gas or charcoal grill . Place breasts on grill, turning them every 4 minutes, for 10 to 12 minutes, or until done. (To check if breasts are done, the meat should be moist and white with no sign of pink when you cut into breast.) Serve hot.

2 medium red peppers

1 medium onion

Place peppers and onions in pan with 2 Tbsp fat-free chicken stock. Sauté until stock is reduced. Spray pan lightly with non-stick cooking oil and sauté another 2 minutes. Salt and pepper to taste.

<u>Serves 4</u>. About 250 Calories per serving (for chicken only).

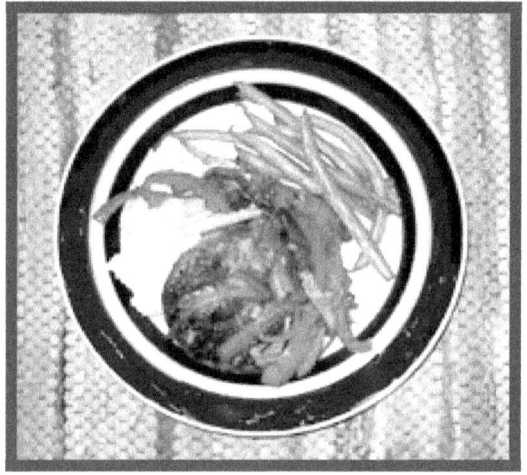

<u>Diet Tip of the Day:</u>. **A reducing diet is best supervised by a physician**. This is especially true when a great deal of weight needs to be lost, or if you have an ailment or a history of medical problems.

Day 4 Recipe
Meat Loaf

½ pound ground white meat turkey
½ pound ground beef (about 90% lean)
1 large egg
½ cup skim milk
¼ cup bread crumbs
¼ cup ketchup
¼ cup chopped carrots
¼ cup chopped onion

In a medium bowl, combine all ingredients. Add salt and pepper to taste. Mix until blended and form into a loaf. Place loaf into oven preheated to 350 °F. Bake until an instant-read thermometer inserted in the center of the loaf reads 160 °F. This should take about one hour.

Shown below is meat loaf, acorn squash baked with 1 tsp maple syrup and steamed spinach drizzled with extra-virgin olive oil (Evoo).

Serves 5. Each serving of meat loaf is about 290 Calories (for meat loaf only).

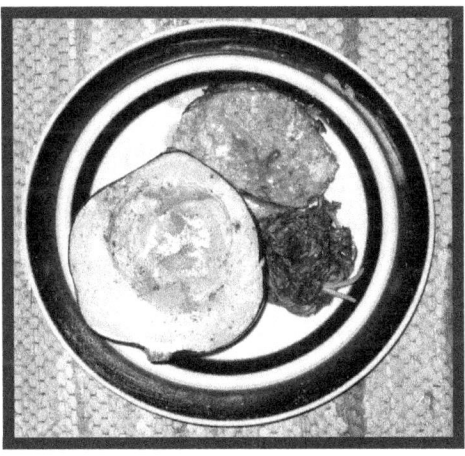

Diet Tip of the Day: Keep a daily food log to record everything you eat. It really does work wonders.

Day 5 Recipe
Frozen-Fish Dinner

No recipe today. No cooking today. It's your day off! To find a frozen fish dinner please go to Appendix A (page 106) which lists approximately 150 frozen dinners manufactured by Healthy Choice, Lean Cuisine and Smart Ones.

Perusing the list, it is obvious that there are not many frozen fish dinners for sale at supermarkets. Note that if you do not use all of the **340 Calories allocated for this Day 5 meal**, use the excess calories anyway you wish. Splurge on extra dessert or save the calories for the next day and have a larger piece of pizza!

Please read the important **Frozen-Food Safety Warning** in Appendix B on page 112.

Diet Tip of the Day: **Buy a pedometer** and start walking. For the average person 2,100 steps amounts to walking about one mile. A Harvard study has shown that 8,000 to 10,000 step per day promote weight loss. And you're not obliged to walk continuously until you accrue all 10,000 steps. Rather, all steps throughout the day to wherever and whenever count toward your daily total. Because 10,000 steps a day may not be achievable by some people, particularly those who are elderly, sedentary, or who have chronic diseases, rather than insisting on a blanket 10,000 steps per day, your initial stepping goal should your baseline steps plus an increment of an additional 2,500 steps. (Your baseline being the number of steps you take in an average day.)

Day 6 Recipe
<u>Grandma's Pizza</u>

The following is a pizza recipe used by my Italian grandmother. She was from a small mountain village located between Rome and Naples.

Pizza dough: To save time use prepared dough, preferably whole wheat. Flour a large cutting board. <u>Divide one pound of prepared pizza dough into four parts</u>. Roll out each dough ball as thin as possible.

Tomato sauce: Sauté ½ small onion, chopped fine, in 1 tsp olive oil. Add two finely chopped garlic cloves, 1½ cups chopped plum tomatoes and ½ tsp chopped fresh oregano. Stir and cook about 5 minutes on a low flame.

Pizza preparation & cooking: On each pizza, spread evenly about ¼ cup of the tomato sauce. Add about ½ ounce of shredded part-skim mozzarella cheese, 1 tsp Parmesan cheese, 3 slices of a Portobello mushroom, some torn fresh basil, and drizzle with Evoo. Put pizzas on a pan and place in 475 °F oven for about 15 to 20 minutes, or until crust is crisp and cheese is just melting. (Freeze left over sauce for use on Day 13.)

<u>Serves 4</u>. Make four pizzas. Each pizza contains about 350 Calories.

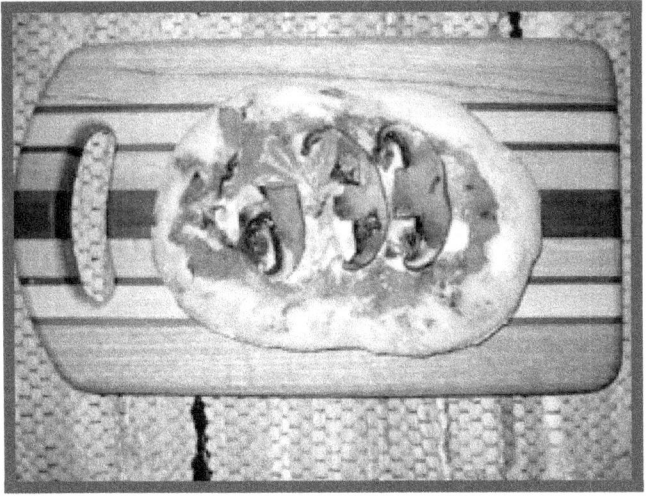

<u>Diet Tip of the Day:</u> For **life-long weight control** take a vigorous 30 to 60 minute walk everyday! That's right – everyday. Make exercise a nonflexible top priority part of your life. When it comes to exercise the key words are consistent, persistent, unyielding, dogged. Get the point?

Day 7 Recipe
<u>Chicken Dinner - Out</u>

No recipe today. No cooking today. Have a chicken dinner at your favorite restaurant, but make sure you choose a restaurant where you have a fighting chance to achieve your calorie goal. Your goal for dinner is a **maximum of 630 Calories**. This includes appetizer, soup, main course and dessert.

Tips for Eating Out: First, order simple, such as broiled chicken breast with steamed vegetables and brown rice. Tell the waiter you want no sauce, no gravy, nothing added. Then, knowing your calorie objective, and that chicken is about 50 Calories per ounce, most steamed vegetable servings average approximately 50 Calories per cup, and rice is about 100 Calories per ½ cup, decide how much to eat – and take the remainder home. If fresh fruit is not an option, pass on dessert and have the evening snack specified for that day in the diet.

In a restaurant, some nutritionists recommend you eat the low-calorie items on your plate first. Start with the salad, soup and veggies. By the time you get to the chicken and starches you will hopefully be full enough to be content with smaller portions of the higher-calorie choices.

Finally, some dieticians advise their dieting clients not to eat out. That's right. They believe eating at home is safer. But our thought is you have to eat out eventually so why not learn how while your resolve is high?

<u>Diet Tip of the Day:</u> When you're on a diet, eating in a restaurant can be a challenge, because most restaurant portions are huge, and can easily total more than 1,000 Calories. When eating in a restaurant decide how much to eat – and take the remainder home. A good general rule of thumb is to **eat half and bring the rest home**.

Day 8 Recipe
Baked Salmon with Salsa

This is a simple, straight-forward recipe. Again, the advantage of a simple recipe is there are no hidden calories.

  4 5 oz salmon fillets
  6 Tbsp bottled tomato-pepper salsa

Brown salmon fillets in non-stick pan and place in baking dish. Put fillets in an oven preheated to 350 °F for about 10 minutes. Plate the salmon. Stir prepared tomato-pepper salsa and spoon it over the salmon.
Serves 4. One salmon fillet is about 215 Calories.

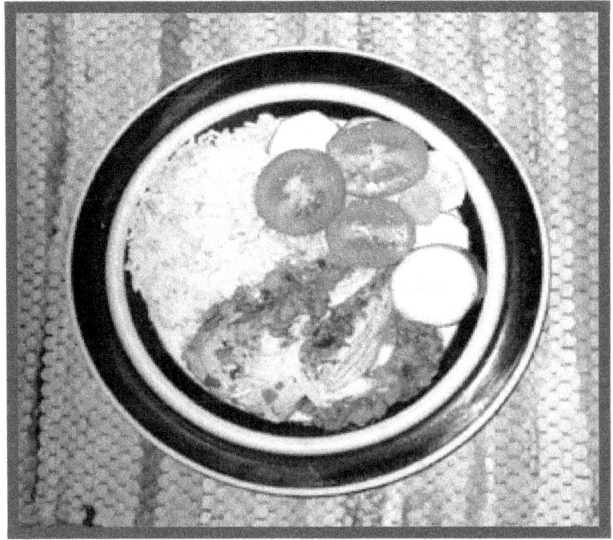

Diet Tip of the Day: **Have soup more often.** Most non-cream-based soups are filling and low-calorie.

Day 9 Recipe
<u>Veggie Burger</u>

Vegetable-based burgers can be purchased at your local supermarket. The patty of a veggie burger can be made from vegetables, soy, nuts, mushrooms, textured vegetable protein, dairy, or a combination of these foods.

Two popular veggie burgers are the Boca Burger and Gardenburger. The Boca Burger is made chiefly from soy protein and wheat gluten. (Boca Burger patties are 2.5 oz each and range from 60 to 90 Calories.) The original Gardenburger is made from mushrooms, onions, brown rice, rolled oats, cheese, and spices. (Gardenburger patties are 2.5 oz each and about 100 Calories.)

To prepare, follow package directions. The version shown below has an added slice of low-fat cheddar cheese. The lettuce, tomato and ketchup shown actually add very few extra calories.

The veggie burger patty plus low-fat cheese amounts to approximately 150 Calories. Add a seeded roll and the total rises to 290 Calories.

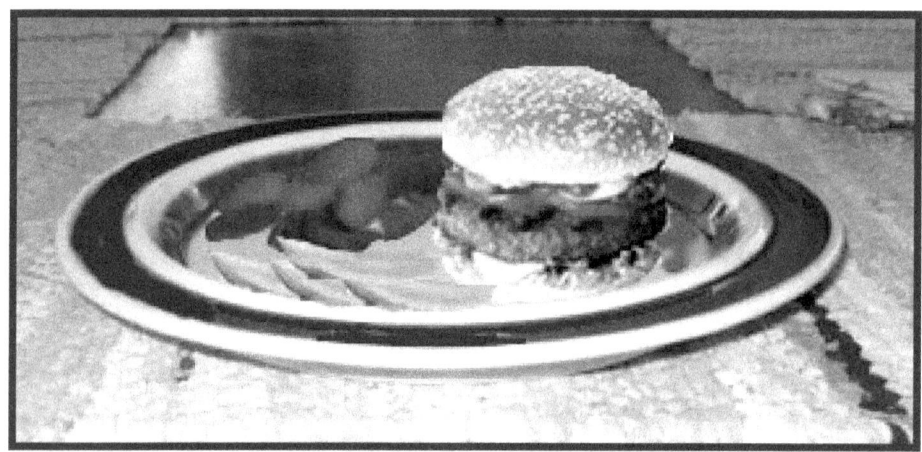

<u>Diet Tip of the Day:</u> **Drink lots of water** – about 8 glasses per day. Add a slice of lemon to make it more interesting. Often, when you think you're hungry, you are just thirsty. So, next time you head for a snack, drink some water first and see if that does it for you.

Day 10 Recipe
<u>Wild Blueberry Pancakes</u>

This recipe makes a relatively low calorie, wholesome batch of delicious wild blueberry-whole wheat-buttermilk pancakes.

   1 cup whole-wheat flour
   1 cup buttermilk
   1 egg
   1 Tbsp vegetable oil
   1 tsp baking powder
   ½ tsp baking soda

Stir ingredients until blended. Add ¾ cup blueberries and gently stir. Using medium heat, preheat a non-stick skillet coated with cooking spray. Pour slightly less than ¼ cup of batter onto skillet per pancake. Cook slowly until bubbles break on surface of pancake. Turn and cook until other side is lightly browned. Makes 8 pancakes.

Pictured below are wild-blueberry pancakes with two slices of turkey bacon.

Serves 4. Each pancake is about 95 Calories

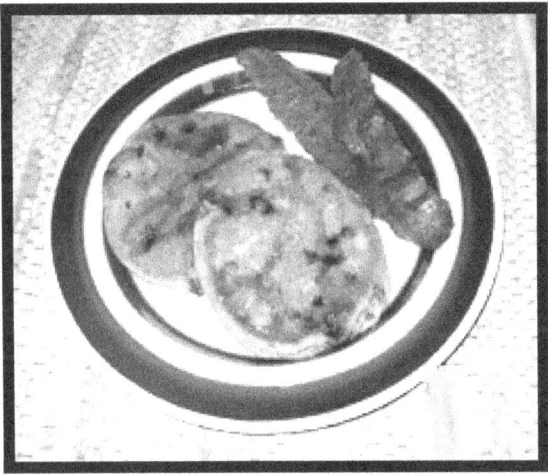

<u>Diet Tip of the Day:</u> A peanut butter sandwich on whole wheat bread with a glass of skim milk and an apple makes a nutritious, reasonably low-calorie lunch.

Day 11 Recipe
<u>Artichoke-Bean Salad</u>

1 can (19 oz) white kidney beans
10 artichoke hearts, quartered
⅓ cup chopped oregano
⅓ cup chopped parsley
3 cloves garlic, chopped
1 lemon, juiced

Combine ingredients in medium-size bowl. Stir in ¼ cup Evoo. Salt and black pepper to taste.

Serves 6. Artichoke-bean salad has approximately 190 Calories per serving.

Pictured on the plate below are two grilled chicken sausage links with salsa, steamed green beans and the artichoke-bean salad. Incidentally, this artichoke-bean combination over mixed salad greens served with a whole-grain bread makes a delicious, nutritious and reasonable low-calorie main course.

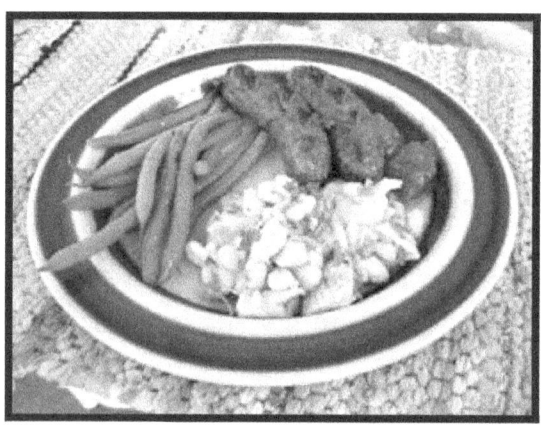

<u>Diet Tip of the Day:</u> Have a small meal before you go to a party. A hardboiled egg, an apple, and a thirst quencher (like water, tea, seltzer, or diet soda) will take the edge off your appetite and make it easier to resist the high-calorie goodies.

Day 12 Recipe
<u>Fish Dinner - Out</u>

No recipe today. No cooking today. Have a fish dinner at your favorite restaurant, but make sure you choose a restaurant where you have a good chance to achieve your calorie goal. For Day 12, your **goal for dinner is a maximum of 595 Calories**. This includes appetizer, soup, main course and dessert.

Tips for Eating Out: The following is almost an exact repeat of advice given for Day 7. First, order simple, such as broiled fish with steamed vegetables and brown rice. Tell the waiter you want no sauce, no gravy, nothing added. Then, knowing your calorie objective, and that fish is about 50 Calories per ounce, most steamed vegetable servings average approximately 50 Calories per cup, and rice is about 100 Calories per ½ cup, decide how much to eat – and take the remainder home. If fresh fruit is not an option, pass on dessert and have the evening snack specified for that day in the diet.

In a restaurant, I recommend you eat the low-calorie items on your plate first. Start with the salad, soup and veggies. By the time you get to the fish and starches you will hopefully be full enough to be content with smaller portions of the higher-calorie choices.

<u>**Diet Tip of the Day:**</u> Phytonutrients are found in plant foods such as fruits, vegetables, whole grains, dried beans, nuts and seeds. Unlike protein, fat, vitamins and minerals, phytonutrients are not necessary for life, but evidence is growing that phytonutrients have many beneficial qualities.

Day 13 Recipe
<u>Pasta with Marinara Sauce</u>

Prepare the sauce as you did for the Day 6 pizza. But because the pizza sauce is a bit too thick, add ¼ cup of pasta liquid to thin it. (The spiral pasta shape shown below is called Fusilli, and is a favorite because all the ridges really hold the sauce.)

½ pound <u>whole-wheat</u> pasta

¼ tsp salt

Prepare the marinara tomato sauce as per Day 6 sauce but dilute it with ¼ cup of pasta liquid. Bring 2 quarts of lightly salted water to a boil. Add pasta and stir occasionally (to keep pasta from sticking to the bottom of the pot). Keep water boiling and cook until pasta are "al dente." (Cooking time is approximately 9 minutes.) Drain pasta, add marinara sauce and serve hot.

Serves 4. One serving is about 225 Calories.

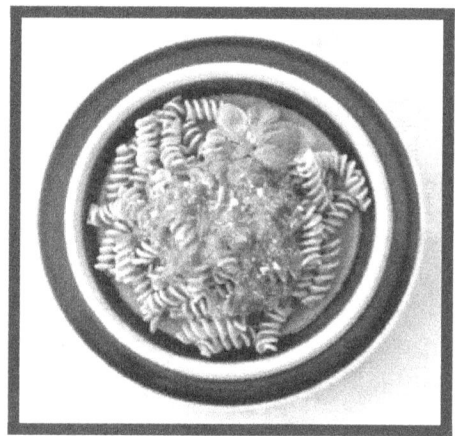

Diet Tip of the Day: **Beware of alcoholic beverages**. Beer has about 13 Calories per ounce, wine 25 Calories per ounce and whiskey 71 Calories per ounce.

Day 14 Recipe
"Oatena" Cereal Mix

Mixing nutritious cereals, hot or cold, is a good way to add variety as well as nutrition to a meal. This recipe features a mix of two whole grain cereals: Oatmeal and Wheatena.

- ⅓ cup Oatmeal
- ¼ cup (4 Tbsp) Wheatena
- ¾ cup water
- ½ cup skim milk
- ¼ cup blueberries
- 10 raisins

Add Oatmeal, Wheatena, raisins and a dash of salt to a microwave-safe cereal bowl. Next add water and stir. Place bowl in microwave, on high power for about 1½ minutes, or until desired consistency is reached. The result is "Oatena," a mix of oatmeal and Wheatena, shown (half eaten) below.

Add skim milk and blueberries and serve hot. Because of the natural sugar in blueberries and raisins, adding sugar is not necessary.

Serves 1. About 310 Calories per serving

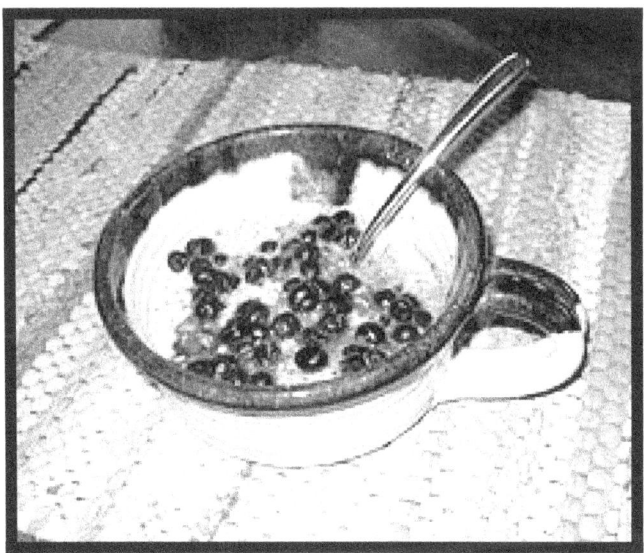

Diet Tip of the Day: Hot or cold cereal topped with fruit, and fat-free milk makes a nutritious, relatively low-calorie meal anytime.

Day 15 Recipe
London Broil

1 pound boneless flank steak about ¾" thick, trimmed of fat

1 clove garlic

1 tsp dry oregano

Rub each side of the flank steak with garlic. Season with oregano, salt and pepper to taste. Prepare a large non-stick skillet over high heat. Steak should sizzle when placed on hot skillet. Sear steak on one side for about 5 minutes; then turn and sear other side for about 4 minutes, or until done to preference. Check the center by making small incision. Carve into ¼-inch slices.

Serves 4. About 320 Calories per serving (for meat only).

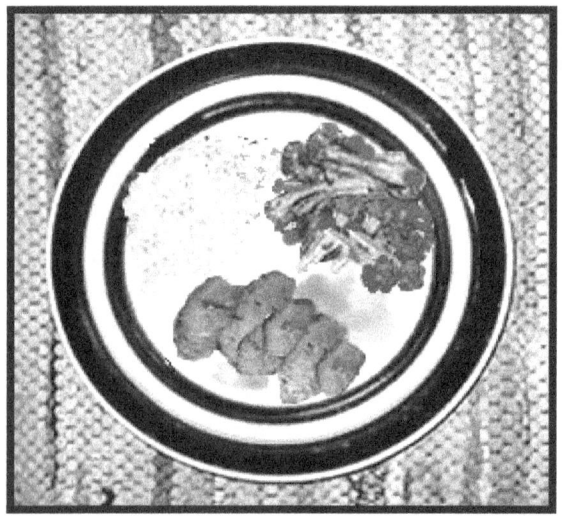

Diet Tip of the Day: **Stay Busy.** Most people will do anything to avoid work, housework, yard work, exercise, etc. But any kind of work burns a lot more calories than just sitting! Whatever it is you are avoiding – just go do it!

Day 16 Recipe
<u>Baked Red Snapper</u>

4 red snapper fillets – 4 oz each (salmon may be substituted)
½ cup white wine
½ cup non-fat yogurt mixed with half as much mustard
½ pound green beans
20 cherry tomatoes
4 tsp olive oil
1 cup wild rice, brown rice and wheat berry mix

Prepare rice mix per package directions.

Brown fillets in non-stick pan. Place fillets skin side down in baking dish coated with non-stick spray. Add white wine and cook in oven preheated to 350 ºF for about 15 minutes. Spoon pan juices over fillets. Salt and pepper to taste.

Place green beans in skillet. Add ¼-inch of water and cook over medium heat until water boils off. Add cherry tomatoes and olive oil. Stir well and sauté for a few minutes. Season with fresh rosemary and oregano. Salt and pepper to taste.

Plate red snapper fillet and spoon over yogurt-mustard sauce. Add green beans & tomato mix and the wild rice. Serve hot.

<u>Serves 4</u>. One plate consisting of one snapper fillet (215 Calories) with green beans & tomato mix (75 Calories) and wild rice (160 Calories) totals 450 Calories.

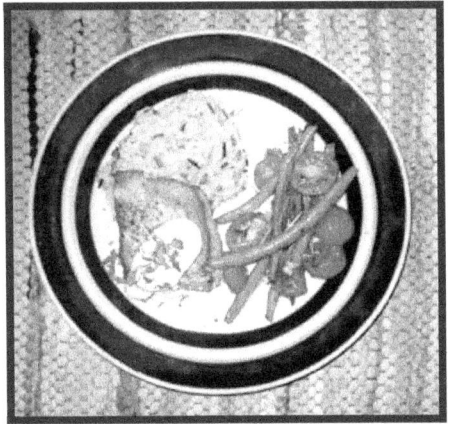

<u>Diet Tip of the Day:</u> **Don't have sweets in your house**. This makes them easier to resist. Out of sight, out of mind!

Day 17 Recipe
Cajun Chicken Salad
This is a perfect after-work, quick, nutritious and delicious dinner.

4 boneless and skinless chicken breasts (about 5 oz each)
1 bottle Cajun spices
8 ounces mixed salad greens
20 cherry tomatoes
12 pitted black olives

Brush chicken breasts lightly with olive oil. Roll breasts in Cajun spices. Brown breasts on non-stick oven-proof skillet. After breasts are brown, put skillet in 350 °F oven for approximately 15 minutes, or until done. Cut breasts into ½-inch slices. (When the breasts are done, the meat should be moist and white with no sign of pink.) Serve hot or keep in an oven or warmer at 200 °F until ready to plate.

Place chicken slices over a bed of mixed salad greens. Add tomatoes, olives and 2 Tbsp of your favorite low-calorie salad dressing.
Serves 4. 330 Calories per serving.

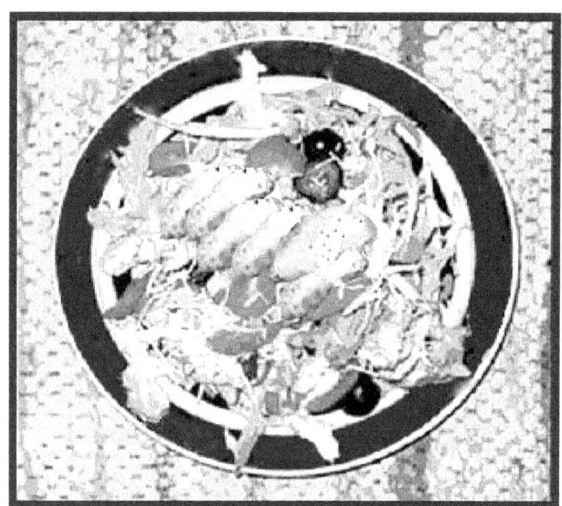

Diet Tip of the Day: Know that **fat-free isn't always your best bet**. Very often sugar is substituted for fat and the calorie total remains the same. Low fat does not necessarily mean low calorie! Rather, look for low-calorie or reduced-calorie products.

Day 18 Recipe
Grilled Swordfish

1¼ pounds swordfish
1 bottle citrus-herb marinade
24 cherry tomatoes
4 medium potatoes
2 cups fresh spinach
1 tsp rosemary & juice of ¼ lemon
2 tsp extra virgin olive oil (Evoo)

Steam spinach with garlic and drizzle with Evoo. Cut up potatoes and place sprinkle with lemon juice, add rosemary, salt and black pepper. Place on grill for about 10 minutes, turning occasionally.

Toss cherry tomatoes in small amount Evoo. Add fresh oregano, salt and black pepper. Place on heavy-duty aluminum foil, seal and grill for about 3 minutes.

Marinade swordfish in citrus-herb vinaigrette. Grill on hot fire for about 5 minutes on one side and 3 minutes on the other, or until done as desired.

Serves 4. One plate consisting of grilled swordfish (250 Calories) with grilled potatoes (100 Calories) and cherry tomatoes (45 Calories) and steamed spinach (50 Calories) totals 445 Calories.

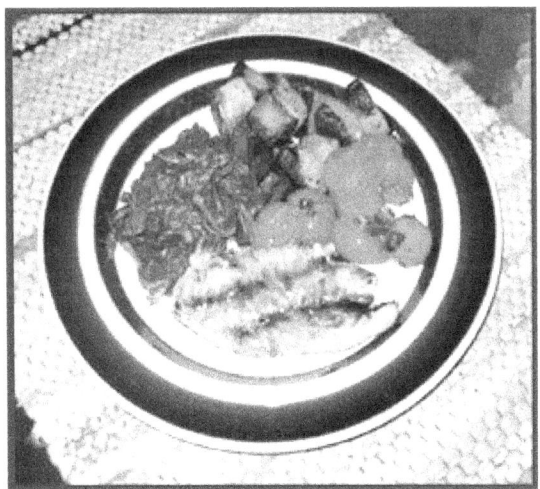

Diet Tip of the Day: Don't be in a hurry to lose weight. Slow weight loss is healthier, is more likely to be permanent, and is easier to sustain over the long haul.

Day 19 Recipe
<u>Chinese Food - Out</u>

No recipe today. No cooking today. Have a Chinese dinner at your favorite restaurant, but make sure you choose a restaurant where you have a reasonable chance to achieve your calorie goal. For today, **your goal for dinner is a maximum of 640 Calories**. This includes any appetizer, soup, main course and any dessert.

Tips for Eating Chinese: You can consume a lot of calories in a Chinese restaurant – if you order carelessly. For example a typical portion of General Tso's chicken is loaded with about 1000 Calories, then add another 200 Calories for a cup of rice.

First rule, order simple. Look for a dish with lots of vegetables, some fish or chicken and brown rice. Tell the waiter you want your food steamed with any sauce on the side. (This is not only a low-calorie way of eating Chinese food but is also the most nutritious way to eat Chinese.)

Then, knowing your 640 Calorie objective, and that chicken and fish are about 50 Calories per ounce, most steamed vegetable servings average approximately 50 Calories per cup, and rice is about 200 Calories per cup, decide how much of the meal you can eat – and take the remainder home. Pass on dessert and have the evening snack specified for that day in the diet. Also see wedge on **Eating Out** (page 10) for more guidance.

<u>Diet Tip of the Day:</u> Another dilemma for dieters is **judging portion size**. It makes no sense to worry about whether to apportion 70 or 80 Calories per ounce for a cut of lean meat if you have no idea whether the portion you are planning to eat weighs four or ten ounces. To be successful, you must learn to estimate portion sizes with reasonable accuracy.

Day 20 Recipe
<u>Quick Pasta alla Puttanesca</u>

This famous pasta dish originated in Naples. Puttanesca means "ladies of the night." The exact origin of the name is unclear, but one thing is clear: It's delicious! Here is one of many recipe versions.

½ pound spaghetti (whole wheat preferred)
20 black pitted olives
1 can (14½ oz) diced tomatoes
½ can (4 oz) tomato sauce
2 Tbsp Evoo
3 cloves of garlic, chopped and 1Tbsp dried minced onion
½ tsp crushed red pepper flakes
1 Tbsp capers drained and rinsed
¼ cup currants

Cook spaghetti according to package directions. Drain and return spaghetti to pot; add a teaspoon Evoo and toss to coat.

Heat 2 tablespoons olive oil in large skillet over medium-high heat. Add red pepper flakes; cook and stir 1 to 2 minutes or until sizzling. Add onion and garlic; cook and stir 1 minute. Finally, add tomatoes with juice, tomato sauce, olives, currants and capers. Cook over medium-high heat, stirring frequently, until sauce is heated through.

<u>Serves 4</u>. About 345 Calories per serving

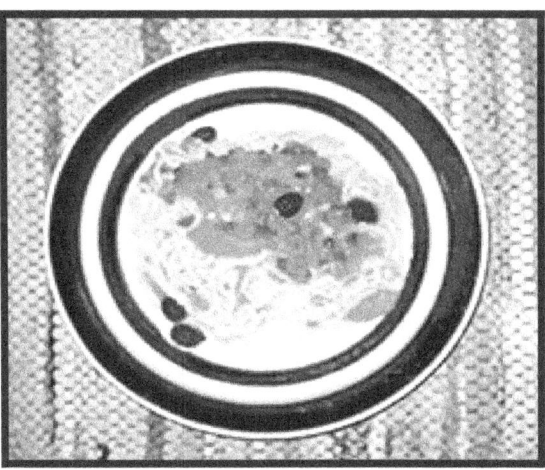

<u>Diet Tip of the Day:</u> Dilute juices, such as apple juice, orange, etc. with water. This cuts the flavor slightly but really reduces calorie content.

Day 21 Recipe
<u>Frozen-Meat Dinner</u>

No recipe today. No cooking today. It's your day off! To find a frozen meat dinner entrée please go to Appendix A (page 106) which lists approximately 150 frozen dinners manufactured by Healthy Choice, Lean Cuisine and Smart Ones.

Note that if you do not use all of the **300 Calories allocated for the Day 21 frozen dinner**, use the excess calories anyway you wish. Splurge on extra dessert or save the calories for another day.

Please read the important **Frozen-Food Safety Warning** in Appendix B on page 112.

<u>**Diet Tip of the Day:**</u> A good understanding of nutrition is not only vital for good health but also will help you control your weight over the long term. For example, did you know that foods that are an "excellent source" of a particular nutrient provide 20% or more of the Recommended Daily Value. Whereas, foods that are a "good source" of a nutrient provide between 10 and 20% of the Recommended Daily Value.

Day 22 Recipe
Shrimp & Spinach Salad

2 pounds shrimp in shell
½ pound small green beans, trimmed
½ pound baby spinach leaves
2 Tbsp lemon juice
¼ cup Evoo
2 tsp minced fresh dill
1 Tbsp minced green onion

To make vinaigrette, combine lemon juice, olive oil, dill, salt and pepper to taste and whisk until blended. Stir in minced onion and set aside.

Peel, de-vein and butterfly shrimp. Place shrimp in a bowl and add water to cover. Add 1 teaspoon of salt, and let stand for 10 minutes. Drain, rinse, drain again, and dry. Arrange shrimp in broiling pan without a rack. Brush shrimp with a little vinaigrette and place under preheated broiler, about 3 inches from heat. Broil about 3 to 4 minutes, turning shrimp once, or until both sides turn pink.

Remove shrimp from broiler and add remaining vinaigrette and green beans to the broiling pan. Stir to coat shrimp and beans with vinaigrette. Pour warm vinaigrette over spinach and toss quickly. Plate the spinach and arrange shrimp and green beans on top.

Serves 4. 310 Calories per serving.

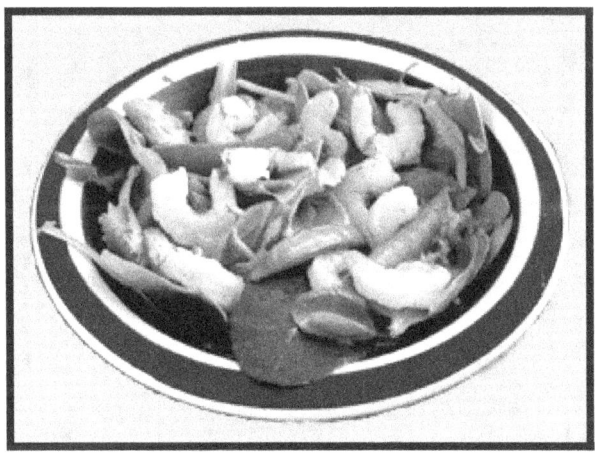

Diet Tip of the Day: After company leaves, have them take some of the leftover food (particularly the dessert) with them – or take the leftovers to work the next day.

Day 23 Recipe
Beans & Greens Salad

⅓ cup chopped oregano
⅓ cup chopped parsley
3 cloves garlic, chopped
1 lemon, juiced

Prepare salad dressing by combining above ingredients and stirring in ¼ cup Evoo. Salt and pepper to taste.

½ pound mesclun mix
¼ pound green beans
1 19 oz can garbanzo beans (chickpeas)

Arrange mesclun mix, garbanzo beans and green beans on a large platter. Drizzle salad dressing over beans and greens.

Serves 4. Approximately 260 Calories per serving.

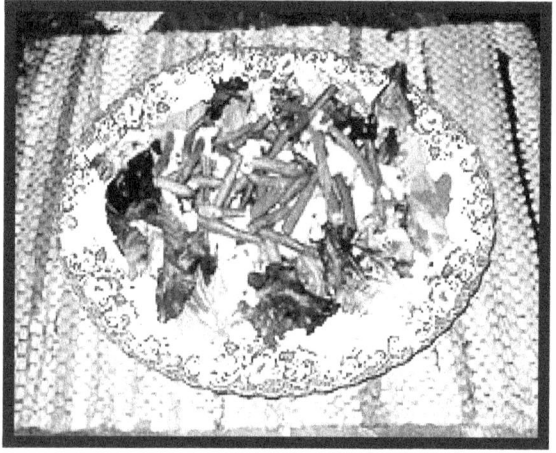

Diet Tip of the Day: Beans are a wonderful food but they are an incomplete protein. If however beans are eaten with a whole-grain bread, the combination forms a complete protein – just as complete and nutritious as meat, poultry, or fish.

Day 24 Recipe
Four-Bean Plus Salad

Note that the total caloric value of the salad will change very little, if the proportions of the bean varieties and corn are varied – according to taste.

½ cup canned red kidney beans, drained and rinsed
½ cup canned black beans, drained and rinsed
½ cup canned chick peas, drained and rinsed
½ cup canned cannelloni beans, drained and rinsed
½ cup canned corn, drained
1 small red pepper, chopped
1 small green pepper, chopped
2 Tbsp Evoo
2 Tbsp lemon juice

In a large bowl mix red kidney beans, black beans, chick peas, cannelloni beans, corn and chopped red and green peppers. Stir in Evoo and lemon juice and plate.

Serves about 6. One serving is ½ cup – with about 135 Calories per serving

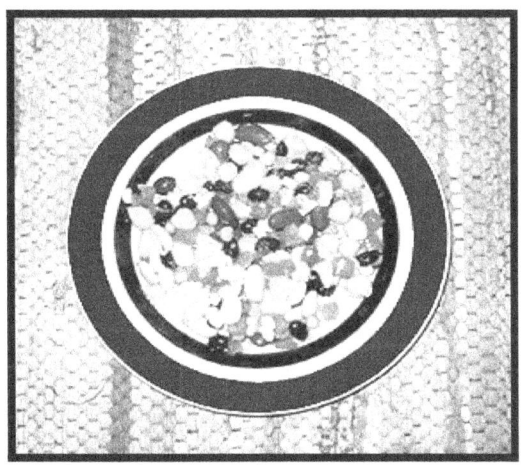

Diet Tip of the Day: Vigorous exercise doesn't necessarily stimulate you to overeat. Just the opposite. In many cases, exercise actually helps curb your appetite – immediately following a workout.

Day 25 Recipe
<u>Pan-Broiled Hanger Steak</u>

1¼ pounds hanger steak, well trimmed of fat

¼ cup lime juice

8 small new potatoes, peeled and halved

12 cherry tomatoes, cut in half

Season both sides of steak with salt and pepper and place in sealable plastic bag with lime juice. Refrigerate for about one hour.

Boil potatoes about 10 minutes. Rinse in cold water. Sauté potatoes in small amount of vegetable oil over medium-high heat until brown.

Sauté cherry tomatoes in small amount of olive oil over medium-high heat until skin begins to crack. Season with chopped fresh basil.

Heat a skillet over medium-high heat. Sear hanger steak on one side for about 5 minutes. Turn over and sear other side approximately 5 minutes (for medium done). Pour off any fat that may have accumulated. Carve into ½-inch slices.

<u>Serves 4.</u> About 320 Calories per serving (for the hanger steak only)

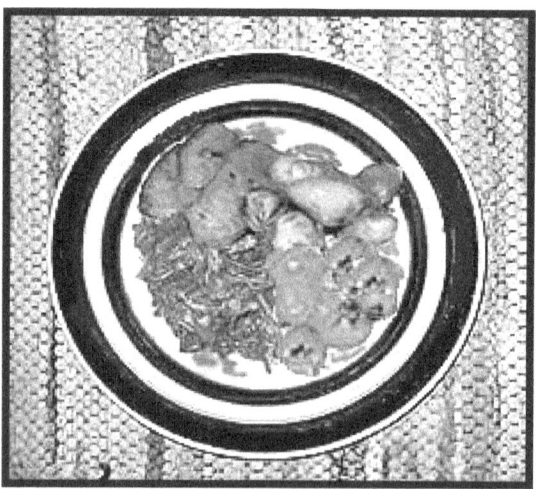

<u>Diet Tip of the Day:</u> If you find yourself at a party, don't stand near the food! Be aware of the temptation. Make the effort, and you'll find you eat less.

Day 26 Recipe
<u>Grilled Scallops and Polenta</u>

1 pound sea scallops
¾ cup polenta cornmeal
¾ cup skim milk
1 medium Portobello mushroom
½ pound green beans
¼ cup chopped red onion
16 asparagus spear
1 tsp Evoo

Bring 1½ cups of water and skim milk to rapid boil. Add salt to taste and slowly add polenta while stirring. Reduce heat. Continue stirring until desired consistency is reached. Pour polenta into lightly greased pan. After polenta has cooled cover and refrigerate. Cut chilled polenta into 4 pieces. Grill on medium-hot fire – about two minutes on each side.

Brush Portobello mushroom and asparagus spear with Evoo and place on grill for about 3 minutes on each side.

Grill scallops on medium-hot fire. Turn after two minutes or when first side turns opaque. Grill until second side turns opaque – about another 2 minutes. Don't overcook but test a scallop by cutting to make sure it's cooked through. Salt and pepper to taste.

<u>Serves 4</u>. The food on the plate pictured below totals 380 Calories.

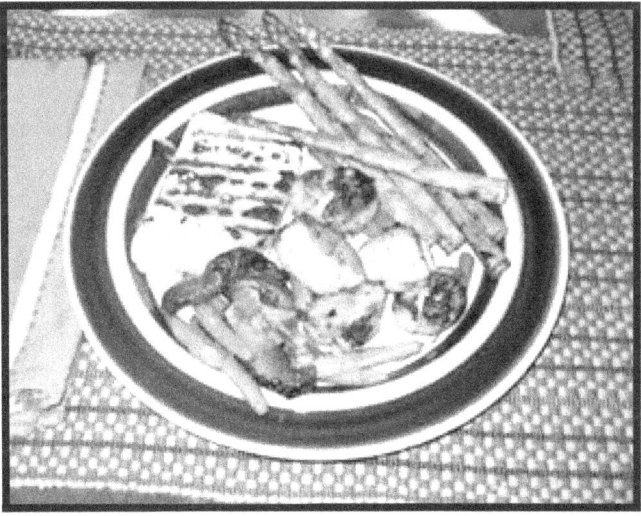

<u>Diet Tip of the Day:</u> To have better control of what you eat **bring your lunch to work**.

Day 27 Recipe
<u>Fettuccine in Summer Sauce</u>

This sauce is often served in the summer because it's lighter than what is usually dished up with pasta. But despite its name the sauce is wonderful year round.

½ pound fettuccine
8 ounces fresh asparagus, trimmed & cut into 2" pieces
20 cherry tomatoes, halved
2 Tbsp plus 1 tsp Evoo
2 cloves of garlic, chopped
½ small onion, diced

Cook fettuccine according to package directions. Drain and return pasta to pot; add a teaspoon Evoo and toss to coat. Meanwhile steam asparagus and drain.

In large skillet over medium-high heat, sauté cherry tomatoes in 2 Tbsp olive oil until skin begins to crack. Add onion and cook until translucent. Stir in garlic . Thin sauce with pasta liquid to desired consistency. Toss cooked pasta and asparagus into sauce and serve immediately.

Serves 4. About 290 Calories per serving

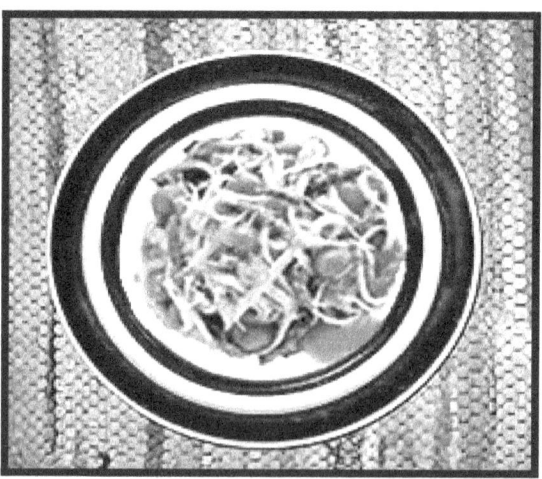

<u>Diet Tip of the Day:</u> A major weight-loss fallacy is that you can get rid of abdominal fat by working your abdominal muscles. This is based on the incorrect belief that fat is eliminated from a particular part of your body if you engage the muscles underneath that layer of fat. No such luck.

Day 28 Recipe
<u>Frozen Chicken MealSm</u>

No recipe today. No cooking today. It's your day off! To find a frozen chicken dinner entrée please go to Appendix A (page 106) which lists approximately 150 frozen dinners manufactured by Healthy Choice, Lean Cuisine and Smart Ones.

Note that if you do not use all of the **300 Calories allocated for the Day 28 frozen dinner**, use the excess calories anyway you wish. Splurge on extra dessert or save the calories for another day.

Please read the important **Frozen-Food Safety Warning** in Appendix B on page 112.

<u>Diet Tip of the Day:</u>   The **general weight-change rule is "last on first off."** Assume as you gained weight, the first place you noticed it was on your thighs, next your buttocks, then your face. As you lose weight, it generally will come off in the reverse order, first from your face, then your rear and finally your thighs. And there is not much you can do about that. The truth is there is no food, no exercise, no magic belt, and no pill that will cause your body to lose fat in one place rather than another.

Day 29 Recipe
Barbequed Shrimp

1½ pounds large shrimp
3 Tbsp bottled barbeque sauce
4 medium ears of corn

Pour barbeque sauce into shallow bowl. Toss shrimp in barbeque sauce to coat. Place shrimp on medium-hot grill. Turn shrimp after about two minutes or when shrimp turn pink. Grill until second side turns pink – approximately another 2 minutes. Don't overcook but test a shrimp by cutting to make sure it is cooked through. Salt and pepper to taste. Serve hot or at room temperature.

Serves 4. About 160 Calories per serving (shrimp only).

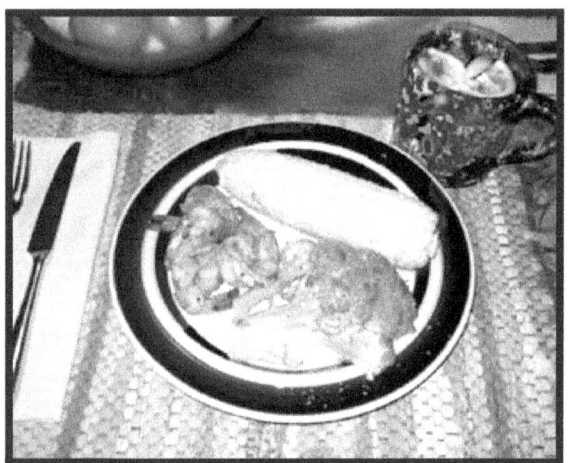

Diet Tip of the Day: A very important weight-profile parameter is your waist-to-hip ratio. Health risks for heart attack and stroke increase considerably for men with a ratio above 1.0 and for women with a ratio above 0.8. To calculate your ratio, measure your waist size (at its narrowest circumference) and divide it by your hip size (at the widest wedge).

Day 30 Recipe

<u>Cheeseburger</u>

There's really not much to grilling hamburgers. The ideal meat for a juicy burger is ground chuck with about 20% fat, but we are talking diet here. So we opt for leaner, much leaner meat.

  1¼ pounds ground sirloin (95% lean)

  4 thin slices low-fat American cheese

Mix ground beef in large bowl. Salt and pepper to taste. Divide into 4 equal portions and form burgers about 1-inch thick. Cook burgers over a hot fire on charcoal or gas-fired grill. For medium, cook about 4 minutes on each side. Top with slice of cheese.

<u>Serves 4</u>. About 320 Calories per serving (hamburger meat only).

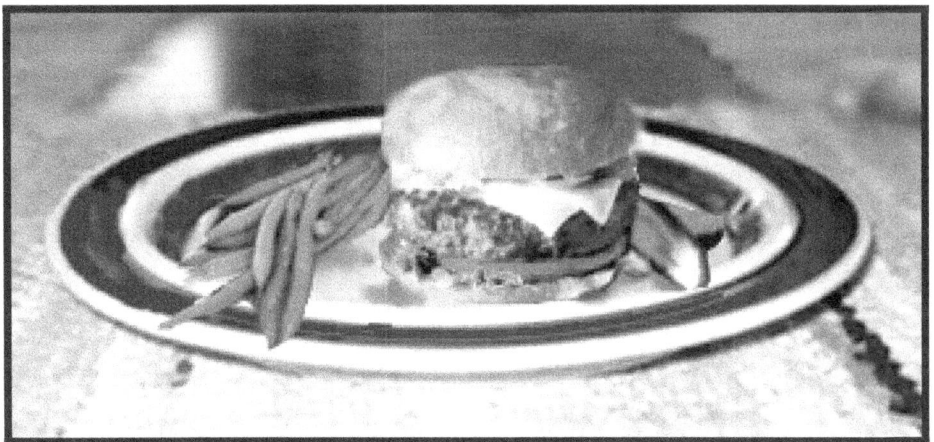

<u>Diet Tip of the Day</u>: Plan to be on a diet the rest of your life. Not necessarily a weight reducing diet. At some point you'll want to just maintain your weight. But you will still need to continue to make good healthy food choices – and not slip back to your old eating habits.

APPENDIX A
Frozen Foods

Appendix A lists three popular brands of frozen entrées: Healthy Choice, Lean Cuisine and Smart Ones. The listing is further divided by entrée type: Poultry entrées, Meat entrées, Seafood entrées, Pasta entrées, Pizza and Other entrées. The entire table is arranged from the lowest to highest in calories. Note that the listed frozen entrées were available in most super markets as of 07/21/2020.

Entrée Type	Name	Brand	Calories
Poultry	Tomato Basil Chicken & Spinach	Smart Ones	160
Meat	Steak Portobella	Lean Cuisine	160
Meat	Asian Style Beef & Broccoli	Smart Ones	~~160~~ 170
Poultry	Herb Roasted Chicken	Lean Cuisine	170
Poultry	Slow Roasted Turkey Breast	Smart Ones	170
Poultry	Grilled Chicken Marsala	Healthy Choice	180
Poultry	Creamy Basil Chicken w Broccoli	Smart Ones	~~180~~ 170
Poultry	Garlic Chicken Rolls	Lean Cuisine	180
Meat	Beef Merlot	Healthy Choice	180
Meat	Homestyle Beef Pot Roast	Smart Ones	180
Poultry	Roasted Turkey & Vegetables	Lean Cuisine	190
Poultry	Chicken & Broccoli Alfredo	Healthy Choice	190
Poultry	Chicken & Vegetable Stir Fry	Healthy Choice	190
Other	Broccoli & Cheddar Roast Potato	Smart Ones	190
Poultry	Crustless Chicken Pot Pie	Smart Ones	~~200~~ 190
Poultry	Buffalo Style Chicken	Lean Cuisine	~~200~~ 190
Poultry	Home Style Chicken & Potatoes	Healthy Choice	200
Pasta	Angel Hair Marinara	Smart Ones	200
Poultry	Salisbury Steak	Smart Ones	200
Meat	Roast Beef & Mashed Potatoes	Smart Ones	~~220~~ 200
Pasta	Primavera Pasta	Smart Ones	210
Poultry	Honey Balsamic Chicken	Healthy Choice	210

Pasta	Ravioli Florentine	Smart Ones	210
Poultry	Cajun Style Chicken & Shrimp	Healthy Choice	220
Pasta	Cheese Ravioli Mushroom Sauce	Smart Ones	230
Poultry	Ranchero Chicken Wrap	Smart Ones	230
Poultry	Lemon Herb Chicken Picante	Smart Ones	230
Pasta	Cheese Ravioli Mushroom Sauce	Smart Ones	230
Meat	Meat Loaf with Mashed Potatoes	Lean Cuisine	~~230~~ 240
Seafood	Shrimp Alfredo	Lean Cuisine	~~230~~ 240
Poultry	Chicken Margherita	Smart Ones	~~220~~ 240
Poultry	Grilled Chicken Caesar	Lean Cuisine	240
Poultry	Honey Glazed Turkey & Potatoes	Healthy Choice	240
Pasta	Spicy Penne Arrabbiata	Lean Cuisine	240
Pasta	Four Cheese Cannelloni	Lean Cuisine	~~240~~ 250
Poultry	Creamy Basil Chicken with Tortellini	Lean Cuisine	~~240~~ 250
Pasta	Cheese Ravioli	Lean Cuisine	250
Pasta	Vermont Cheddar Mac & Cheese	Lean Cuisine	250
Pasta	Fettuccini Alfredo	Smart Ones	250
Poultry	Oriental Chicken	Smart Ones	250
Poultry	Fiesta Grilled Chicken	Lean Cuisine	250
Pasta	Chicken Linguini Red Pepper	Healthy Choice	250
Poultry	Golden Roasted Turkey Breast	Healthy Choice	250
Poultry	Chicken Mesquite	Smart Ones	250
Poultry	Chicken Oriental	Smart Ones	250
Poultry	Orange Sesame Chicken	Smart Ones	250
Poultry	Baked Chicken	Lean Cuisine	~~250~~ 260
Poultry	Teriyaki Chicken & Vegetables	Smart Ones	~~250~~ 260
Seafood	Tuna Noodle Casserole	Smart Ones	~~250~~ 270
Pasta	Spaghetti with Meatballs	Lean Cuisine	260
Poultry	Creamy Chicken & Noodles	Healthy Choice	260
Meat	Barbecue Steak w Red Potatoes	Healthy Choice	260

Pasta	Tortellini Primavera Parmesan	Healthy Choice	260
Pasta	Sesame Noodles with Vegetables	Smart Ones	~~260~~ 280
Pasta	Creamy Rigatoni w Chicken	Smart Ones	260
Pasta	Macaroni & Cheese	Smart Ones	260
Pasta	Butternut Squash Ravioli	Lean Cuisine	260
Other	Santa Fe Rice & Beans	Smart Ones	260
Other	Coconut Chickpea Curry	Lean Cuisine	260
Poultry	Glazed Turkey Tenderloins	Lean Cuisine	270
Poultry	Kung Pao Chicken	Healthy Choice	270
Poultry	Chicken Margherita w Balsamic	Healthy Choice	270
Poultry	Chicken Strips & Sweet Potatoes	Smart Ones	270
Pasta	Spaghetti with Meat Sauce	Smart Ones	~~270~~ 280
Meat	Salisbury Steak with Mac & Cheese	Lean Cuisine	~~270~~ 290
Pasta	Penne Rosa	Lean Cuisine	270
Poultry	Turkey Breast & Stuffing	Smart Ones	~~270~~ 280
Pasta	Classic Macaroni & Beef	Lean Cuisine	270
Pasta	Mushroom Mezzaluna Ravioli	Lean Cuisine	270
Pasta	Pasta with Swedish Meatballs	Smart Ones	~~280~~ 290
Other	Asian Pot Stickers	Lean Cuisine	280
Poultry	Sesame Stir Fry with Chicken	Lean Cuisine	280
Poultry	Roasted Turkey Breast	Lean Cuisine	~~280~~ 290
Poultry	Apple Cranberry Chicken	Lean Cuisine	280
Poultry	Chicken Fettuccini Alfredo	Healthy Choice	280
Poultry	Grilled Chicken Marinara	Healthy Choice	280
Poultry	Sweet & Spicy Orange Chicken	Healthy Choice	280
Poultry	Chicken Parmesan	Smart Ones	280
Poultry	Turkey Breast with Stuffing	Smart Ones	280
Meat	Beef & Broccoli	Healthy Choice	280
Meat	Meatball Marinara	Healthy Choice	280

Meat	Beef Teriyaki	Healthy Choice	280
Pasta	Spinach Artichoke Ravioli	Lean Cuisine	280
Other	Vegetable Fried Rice	Smart Ones	280
Pasta	Spinach Artichoke Ravioli	Lean Cuisine	280
Pasta	Linguini with Ricotta & Spinach	Lean Cuisine	280
Poultry	Chicken Fettuccini	Lean Cuisine	~~290~~ 280
Pasta	Spaghetti & Meatballs	Healthy Choice	280
Pasta	Spaghetti with Meat Sauce	Smart Ones	280
Other	Vegetable Fried Rice	Smart Ones	280
Other	Asian Pot Stickers	Lean Cuisine	280
Poultry	Chicken with Almonds	Lean Cuisine	290
Poultry	Chicken with Peanut Sauce	Lean Cuisine	290
Seafood	Shrimp & Angel Hair Pasta	Lean Cuisine	~~280~~ 290
Poultry	Grilled Chicken Pesto w Veggies	Healthy Choice	290
Poultry	General Tso's Spicy Chicken	Healthy Choice	290
Poultry	Pineapple Chicken	Healthy Choice	290
Poultry	Chicken Enchiladas Suiza	Smart Ones	290
Meat	Swedish Meatballs	Lean Cuisine	290
Seafood	Lemon Pepper Fish	Healthy Choice	290
Pasta	Pasta with Swedish Meatballs	Smart Ones	290
Other	Santa Fe Rice & Beans	Smart Ones	290
Pizza	Thin Crust Cheese Pizza	Smart Ones	290
Seafood	Parmesan Crusted Fish	Lean Cuisine	~~290~~ 300
Pasta	Santa Fe-Style Rice & Beans	Lean Cuisine	~~280~~ 300
Poultry	Roasted Turkey & Vegetables	Lean Cuisine	~~290~~ 300
Poultry	Sweet & Sour Chicken	Lean Cuisine	300
Poultry	Crustless Chicken Pot Pie	Healthy Choice	300
Poultry	Sweet Sesame Chicken	Healthy Choice	300
Poultry	Chicken Fettuccini	Smart Ones	300
Poultry	General Tso's Chicken	Smart Ones	300

Meat	Classic Meat Loaf	Healthy Choice	300
Seafood	Tortilla Crusted Fish	Lean Cuisine	~~300~~ 310
Pasta	Tuscan-Style Vegetable Lasagna	Lean Cuisine	~~300~~ 310
Pasta	Tortellini with Red Pepper Sauce	Lean Cuisine	300
Pasta	Broccoli Cheddar Rotini	Lean Cuisine	300
Pasta	Three Cheese Ziti Marinara	Smart Ones	300
Pasta	Lasagna Florentine	Smart Ones	~~310~~ 300
Seafood	Tortilla Crusted Fish	Lean Cuisine	~~300~~ 310
Pasta	Tuscan-Style Vegetable Lasagna	Lean Cuisine	~~300~~ 310
Poultry	Chicken Fried Rice	Lean Cuisine	~~300~~ 310
Poultry	Orange Chicken	Lean Cuisine	310
Poultry	Chicken Tikka Masala	Lean Cuisine	310
Poultry	Chicken Strips & Fries	Smart Ones	310
Poultry	Chicken Teriyaki	Lean Cuisine	310
Pizza	Thin Crust Pepperoni Pizza	Smart Ones	310
Pasta	Three Cheese Macaroni	Smart Ones	310
Pizza	French Bread Pepperoni Pizza	Lean Cuisine	310
Poultry	Chicken Spinach Mushroom Panini	Lean Cuisine	~~350~~ 310
Other	Spicy Beef & Bean Enchilada	Lean Cuisine	310
Poultry	Chicken Fried Rice	Healthy Choice	320
Meat	Sweet & Spicy Korean Beef	Lean Cuisine	320
Pizza	Farmers Market Pizza	Lean Cuisine	320
Pizza	Margherita Pizza	Lean Cuisine	320
Poultry	Chicken Carbonara	Lean Cuisine	330
Poultry	Mango Chicken w Coconut Rice	Lean Cuisine	330
Poultry	Country Fried Chicken	Healthy Choice	330
Other	Cheese & Fire-Roasted Tamale	Lean Cuisine	330
Poultry	Chicken Club Panini	Lean Cuisine	~~350~~ 340
Meat	Philly Style Steak and Cheese Panini	Lean Cuisine	~~330~~ 350
Poultry	Chicken Parmigana	Healthy Choice	360

Poultry	Chicken Pecan	Lean Cuisine	~~320~~ 370
Poultry	Sweet & Sour Chicken	Healthy Choice	390
Pizza	Supreme Pizza	Lean Cuisine	~~330~~ 390

APPENDIX B
Frozen Food Safety

Increasingly, food giants like ConAgra, Nestlé and others that supply Americans with processed foods concede that they cannot ensure the safety of their food products. Frozen foods pose a particularly serious safety problem because unsuspecting consumers buy frozen foods for their convenience and incorrectly believe that cooking frozen foods is a matter of taste – not safety.

Still the food industry says that extensive outbreaks of food-borne illness are rare, even though it is well-known that most of the millions of cases of food-borne illness every year go unreported or are not traced to the source. For example, each year approximately 40,000 cases of salmonella poisoning are reported in the United States – but perhaps as many as one million cases go unreported. (Salmonella is a type of bacteria most often found in poultry, eggs, unprocessed milk, meat and water.) Recently salmonella pathogens in some frozen meals have sickened thousands of people. How could this happen? First, the supply chain for ingredients in processed foods – from flour to fruits and vegetables to flavorings – is becoming more complex and global in the drive to keep food costs down. As a result, government and industry officials concede that almost every food ingredient is now a potential carrier of pathogens. A further complication is that a large number of food companies subcontract processing work to save money and don't require suppliers to test for pathogens. In fact, companies often don't even know who is supplying their ingredients.

In addition, many frozen-food manufacturers have stopped cooking their products at high temperatures, a tactic they call the "kill step," which is intended to eliminate any lingering microbes. Frequently this process step turns some of the frozen food ingredients into mush. So, instead the "kill step" has been shifted to consumers. For example, ConAgra has added food safety instructions to its frozen meals, including the Healthy Choice brand. A typical "frozen-food safety" instruction offers this guidance: "Internal temperature needs to reach 165°F as measured by a food thermometer in several spots."

Moreover, General Mills, now advises consumers to avoid microwaves altogether and cook their frozen pizzas only in a conventional oven. **Bottom line**: To be safe, always cook frozen foods so that the internal temperature reaches 165°F as measured by a good food thermometer.

Appendix C
Soup Selections

When the Daily Meal Plan menu specifies soup have only one serving (8 ounces) unless stated otherwise. Note that the listed soups were available in most supermarkets as of 07/21/2020. *These are canned soup selections.

Soup Description	Calories
Healthy Choice Chicken with Rice	90
Campbell's Tomato	100
Healthy Choice Country Vegetable	100
Progresso Minestrone*	110
Progresso Chickarina*	110
Progresso Italian-Style Wedding*	120
Campbell's Home-Style Light Chicken Corn Chowder*	120
Campbell's Home-Style Chicken Noodle	130
Campbell's Home-Style Butter Nut Squash*	130
Campbell's Healthy Request Vegetable Beef	140
Progresso Lentil*	140
Progresso Green Split Pea*	150
Campbell's Slow Kettle New England Clam Chowder	160
Progresso Macaroni and Bean*	160
Progresso New England Clam Chowder*	170
Progresso Lasagna-Style*	170
Progresso Broccoli Cheese with Bacon*	180
As an alternative, have 2 servings of a 90 Cal soup	180
Campbell's Chunky Classic Chicken Noodle	190
Amy's Rustic Italian Vegetable*	190
Campbell's Chunky Beef n Cheese*	200
Amy's French Country Vegetable*	210
Campbell's Chunky Sirloin Burger + Vegetables	220
Enjoy two servings of a 110 or 120 Calorie soup	230
Enjoy two servings of a 120 Calorie soup	240

NoPaperPress eBooks and Paperbacks

100-Day Super Diet-1200 Cal*
100-Day Super Diet-1500 Cal*
100-Day No-Cooking Diet-1200 Cal*
100-Day No-Cooking Diet-1500 Cal*
90-Day Smart Diet-1200 Cal*
90-Day Smart Diet-1500 Cal*
90-Day No-Cooking Diet - 1200 Cal*
90-Day No-Cooking Diet - 1500 Cal*
90-Day Perfect Diet - 1200 Cal*
90-Day Perfect Diet - 1500 Cal*
60-Day Perfect Diet-1200 Cal*
60-Day Perfect Diet-1500 Cal*
50-Day Flex Diet-1200 Cal*
50-Day Flex Diet-1500 Cal*
30-Day Quick Diet - Women*
30-Day Quick Diet for Men*
30-Day No-Cooking Diet*
30-Day Diet - Women - Metric*
30-Day Diet for Men - Metric*
25 Day Easy Diet-1200 Cal*
25 Day Easy Diet-1500 Cal*
25-Day No-Cooking Diet
10-Day Express Diet
10-Day No-Cooking Diet*
7-Day Diet for Women*
7-Day Diet for Men*
7-Day No-Cooking Diets*
90-Day Gluten-Free Diet-1200 Cal*
90-Day Gluten-Free Diet-1500 Cal*
30-Day Gluten-Free Quick Diet*
30-Day Gluten-Free No-Cooking Diet*
7-Day Diet for Women - Metric*
7-Day Diet for Men - Metric
7-Day Gluten-Free Express Diet*
7-Day Gluten-Free No-Cooking Diet*
90-Day Vegetarian Diet-1200 Cal*
90-Day Vegetarian Diet-1500 Cal*
30-Day Vegetarian Diet*
7-Day Vegetarian Diet*
Weight Loss for Women*
Weight Loss for Women - Metric
Weight Loss for Women - UK
Weight Loss for Men*
Maximum Weight Loss - 1200 Cal*
Maximum Weight Loss - 1500 Cal*

Weight Loss for Men - Metric*
Maximum Weight Loss- 1200 Cal*
Maximum Weight Loss- 1500 Cal*
Weight Control - U.S. Edition*
Weight Control - Metric. Edition
Prof Weight Control Women - U.S.
Prof Weight Control Women - Metric
Prof Weight Control Men - U.S.
Prof Weight Control Men - Metric
Weight Maintenance - U.S. Ed*
Weight Maintenance - Metric. Ed*
Weight Maintenance - UK Ed
Weight Loss for Senior Men*
Weight Loss for Senior Women*
Eat Smart - U.S. Edition*
Eat Smart - Metric Edition
30-Day Mediterranean Diet
Exercise Smart - U.S. Edition*
Exercise Smart - Metric Edition
Exercise Smart - UK Edition*
Total Fitness - U.S. Edition
Total Fitness - Metric Edition
Total Fitness - UK Edition
Total Fitness for Women-U.S. Ed*
Total Fitness for Women - Metric
Total Fitness for Women - UK Ed
Total Fitness for Men - U.S. Ed*
Total Fitness for Men- Metric Ed*
Total Fitness for Men - UK Ed
Senior Fitness - U.S. Edition*
Senior Fitness - Metric Edition*
Senior Fitness - UK Edition*
Computer Diet - U.S. Edition*
Computer Diet - Metric Ed*
Reliable Weight Loss - U.S. Ed
101 Weight Loss Tips*
101 Healthy Eating Tips*
101 Lifelong Fitness Tips*
101 Weight Maintenance Tips
101 Weight Loss Recipes
101 GF Weight Loss Recipes
101 Veggie Weight Loss Recipes*
30-Day Mediterranean Diet*
90-Day Med Diet - 1200 Cal*
90-Day Med Diet - 1500 Cal*

* These titles are available as both ebooks and paperbacks. Our ebooks are sold by Amazon, Apple, Google, Barnes & Noble and Kobo, but our paperbacks are only sold by Amazon.

Disclaimer

This book offers general meal planning, nutrition and weight control information. It is not a medical manual and the author does not claim to be medically qualified. The material in this book is not intended to be a substitute for medical counseling. Everyone should have a medical checkup before beginning a weight loss program Moreover, the physician conducting the medical exam should be made aware of and should approve the specific weight control program planned. Additionally, while the author and publisher have made every effort to ensure the accuracy of the information in this book, they make no representations or warranties regarding its accuracy or completeness. Further, neither the author nor publisher assume liability for any medical problems that might result from applying the methods in this book, or for any loss of profit, or any other commercial damages, including but not limited to special, incidental, consequential or other damages, and any such liability is hereby expressly disclaimed.

www.ingramcontent.com/pod-product-compliance
Lightning Source LLC
Chambersburg PA
CBHW060414290526
45791CB00002B/752